Cannabinoids - Recent Perspectives and Applications in Human Health

Edited by Steven P. James

Published in London, United Kingdom

Cannabinoids - Recent Perspectives and Applications in Human Health
http://dx.doi.org/10.5772/intechopen.100996
Edited by Steven P. James

Contributors
Peter Galettis, John Barlow, Jaroslav Boublik, Stefania Capra, Rachel Galettis, Myfanwy Graham, Courtney Hill, Paul Mavor, Jasminka Nikolajevic-Sarunac, Rosemary Richards, Janet Schloss, Melinda Thompson, Linda Truong, Berzenn Urbi, Katrina Weston-Green, Aaron K. Wong, Peter B. Chase, Ali E. Dabiri, Ghassan S. Kassab, Weston J. Umstead, Richard Holdman, Marcelo Einicker-Lamas, Gloria M.R.S. Grelle, Luzia S. Sampaio

First published in London, United Kingdom, 2023 by IntechOpen
IntechOpen is the global imprint of INTECHOPEN LIMITED, registered in England and Wales, registration number: 11086078, 5 Princes Gate Court, London, SW7 2QJ, United Kingdom

British Library Cataloguing-in-Publication Data
A catalogue record for this book is available from the British Library

Additional hard and PDF copies can be obtained from orders@intechopen.com

Cannabinoids - Recent Perspectives and Applications in Human Health
Edited by Steven P. James
p. cm.
Print ISBN 978-1-80356-578-1
Online ISBN 978-1-80356-579-8
eBook (PDF) ISBN 978-1-80356-580-4

Meet the editor

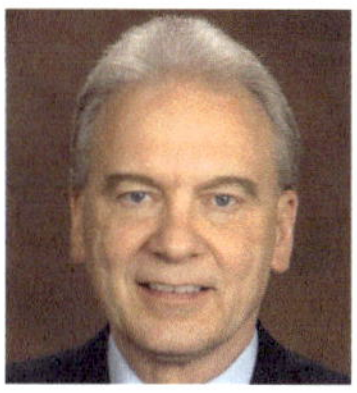

Dr. Steven P. James is the founder of Steven P. James, MD INC, a medical education consulting group focused on providing medical education on topics of neuroscience and cannabinoids. He is also co-founder and chief medical officer (CMO) of Clarity Telehealth, a company dedicated to improving access to patient care and educating healthcare providers and their patients on mental health. He is a medical author and writer and recently published *The Clinicians Guide to Cannabinoid Science*. He has almost three decades of experience as a physician-executive in the pharmaceutical industry. In addition, he is a frequent presenter to both healthcare professionals and the public on topics related to the science of cannabinoids, psychopharmacology, and medical history. He has appeared on ABC's *Good Morning America* and local television and radio programs. Dr. James was born and raised in Owensboro, KY, USA, and attended the University of Kentucky (UK), where he obtained a BS and MD in 1979. He received an MBA from the University of California, Irvine in 1994. He completed his psychiatry residency at New York Presbyterian Hospital (Cornell), a fellowship in psychopharmacology at Stanford University, and a clinical fellowship in psychobiology at the National Institute of Mental Health (NIMH). He subsequently served as Assistant Professor of Psychiatry and cofounder of the Penn Center for Sleep Disorders at the University of Pennsylvania, USA. Currently, he is on the voluntary faculty of psychiatry in the UK. In the pharmaceutical industry, Dr. James has worked in drug development, medical affairs, and global business units for more than 30 years at several companies including Eli Lilly, Elan, Allergan (now AbbVie), Shire, and Merck-Serono. After retiring from the pharmaceutical industry, Dr. James has continued to pursue his career-long interests in improving patient access to mental health, advancing scientific innovation into clinical treatment, and integrating psychiatry into mainstream medical practice. Dr. James is a distinguished fellow and board-certified in the American Board of Psychiatry and Neurology (Psychiatry) and a lifetime fellow of the American Board of Sleep Medicine (ABSM).

Contents

Preface

My interest in cannabinoids and their potential benefit in health care did not arise in medical school, residency, fellowships, or my subsequent clinical work. Only after working for two decades as a physician-scientist in the pharmaceutical industry did I become aware of the importance of cannabinoids in maintaining health and homeostasis. I was intrigued by the scientific evidence suggesting cannabinoids are beneficial for a variety of poorly treated medical conditions. And I was disappointed with how limited this knowledge about cannabinoids was in the general medical community. For healthcare professionals, learning should be a lifetime pursuit built on the foundation of their scientific training. Unfortunately, many clinicians were never exposed to the established scientific data or therapeutic potential of cannabinoids. In general, they have concerns about mental health and addiction from the use of cannabis. At the same time, the public acceptance of cannabis as a potential treatment option is growing rapidly along with the perception (not always warranted) of safety.

It is evident an urgent need exists for additional education about the evolving areas of scientific discovery and the current uses of cannabinoids. I am delighted to serve as editor of *Cannabinoids - Recent Perspectives and Applications in Human Health* and expect this book to address these twin needs and provide both an interesting introduction to developing areas of research and a timely update on clinical applications.

It seems as if everyone (layperson and healthcare professional) is now aware that cannabinoids are naturally occurring compounds found in plants like hemp and cannabis. Most of the earlier interest in cannabinoids from medical scientists, however, was related to their dramatic disruptions of mental health and concerns about tolerance and addiction. Absent was the knowledge about the molecular basis that produced the positive and negative effects of cannabinoids. Finally, in the late twentieth century, the beginning of a revolution in cannabinoid research arrived. Research began to uncover the structure of cannabinoids, leading to unexpected findings about their effects on the human body and their role in human health and disease.

It is established that cannabinoids from plants influence the human body through the Endocannabinoid System (ECS). This breakthrough discovery was a groundbreaking moment in cannabinoid science and revealed the presence of an entire system within the human body previously unsuspected. The ECS is a major regulator of homeostasis in the human body and consists of endocannabinoids, receptors, and enzymes that modulate various physiological processes in the body. The cannabinoids interact with the cannabinoid receptors that are found throughout the central and peripheral nervous systems and modulate neural activity and neurotransmission. Cannabinoids also act on other systems such as the digestive system, immune system, and cardiovascular system. Studies have found that cannabinoids can reduce inflammation, improve pain modulation and neuroprotection, modulate gene expression and metabolism, increase appetite, regulate moods and emotions, help treat certain types of cancer, and may even protect against neurodegenerative diseases. Research continues to discover new ways cannabinoids can be used for therapeutic purposes. At the center of this research is the ECS, which promises to revolutionize how cannabinoids are used for medical purposes.

The legalization of cannabis and the greater social acceptance of marijuana has unexpectedly led to more clinical research into the potential benefits of this plant. Much of this new research has been driven by serendipitous clinical observations about how cannabis helped people in ways that were not necessarily expected. These anecdotal reports of people benefiting from the use of cannabis and these stories have been around for a long time and clinical research is needed to determine if these effects can be reliably reproduced and whether they translate into clinical benefits.

In the past two decades, more than 25,000 articles about cannabinoids have been published in the peer-reviewed medical literature. It would be fair to say that during this recent period, cannabinoids have finally been studied more rigorously than at any other time in history. This scientific curiosity about cannabinoids has been fed by multiple and often unrelated research studies. In this publication, we hope to significantly add to this body of knowledge and encourage the clinician and researcher to do additional activities. One important consequence of this effort is the recent approval by regulatory agencies after a review of well-conducted randomized clinical trials of plant-based Epidiolex and Sativex, which further normalizes the use of cannabinoids in the medical field.

The recent approval of Epidiolex, a cannabidiol (CBD)-based prescription drug, has been an exciting development in the world of cannabinoids. CBD is a non-psychoactive cannabinoid that has shown great potential as a therapeutic agent for two rare forms of epilepsy. The FDA and EMA approval of Epidiolex marks the first time a plant-based cannabinoid has been approved for medical use in the United States and Europe and is available to the patient by prescription filled at the pharmacy.

The approval of Epidiolex has been an exciting development and will pave the way for further research into CBD's potential and the medical applications of other plant-based cannabinoids. With the approval of Epidiolex, further, CBD research is expected to gain momentum in both the United States and Europe.

The FDA and EMA approval of Epidiolex marks the first time a plant-based cannabinoid has been approved for medical use in the United States. As a result of the decriminalization of Cannabinoids, other CBD products can now be studied although these molecules may have significant differences in quality and safety when compared to the approved CBD Epidiolex.

As a result, CBD products can vary greatly in quality and do not have the same safety and efficacy data that Epidiolex has.

Sativex is a second plant-based cannabinoid combination product first approved in the United Kingdom in 2010. It is now currently approved in twenty-nine countries for the treatment of adult patients with moderate-to-severe spasticity due to multiple sclerosis who have not responded adequately to other anti-spasticity medications.

However, the FDA has not approved Sativex for use in the United States due to concerns about its safety and efficacy. The FDA also expressed concern that Sativex could be abused or misused, as it contains psychoactive tetrahydrocannabinol (THC).

These approvals have led to increased acceptance of cannabinoid-based treatments as well as greater public awareness about their potential uses. This has opened a new world of treatment possibilities for patients who are often untreatable by traditional medications. Ultimately, randomized controlled trials will provide a more comprehensive picture of the use of cannabinoids in medicine, making them much more accessible and applicable for healthcare professionals and patients. This process will be especially important for cannabinoids to assume a greater role in clinical practice, as it will provide additional strong and credible science about the safety and benefits of therapies. By establishing the road forward for new plant-based cannabinoids, we will then enter an even more exciting phase in the world of cannabinoids.

As new research comes out, this book will serve as an invaluable resource for a variety of healthcare professionals – from medical doctors and pharmacists to nurses and allied healthcare providers – to further the knowledge necessary for quality care. It is our hope that this book will equip these professionals with the necessary information to navigate the field of cannabinoids and their potential clinical applications to best serve their patients. We believe this book will be instrumental in furthering the understanding of healthcare professionals regarding cannabinoids while also providing an updated resource that they can turn to as new research emerges.

I would like to acknowledge the diligent and always pleasant support of Author Service Manager Tea Jurcic at IntechOpen. Without her constant encouragement, this book would never have been completed.

Steven P. James, MD
Independent Researcher,
Rancho Santa Fe, CA, USA

Section 1

The Science of Cannabinoids

Chapter 1

Polysaccharide Chiral Stationary Phases for the Achiral and Chiral Separation of Cannabinoids

Weston J. Umstead

Abstract

Polysaccharide-based chiral stationary phases (CSPs) have been widely utilized in the pharmaceutical, agricultural, and natural product industries since their first-reported use and subsequent commercialization more than 50 years ago. Although they have been traditionally used for the separation of small drug molecules containing one or more chiral centers, their uses have recently grown to include achiral separations in emerging fields like the cannabis industry. The ability to separate and study individual cannabinoids is critical to understanding their impact in both medicinal and recreational applications. Furthermore, it is not difficult to envision a future where cannabinoids, particularly for medicinal use, are treated like pharmaceuticals—that is requiring rigorous purity testing, including the determination of chiral purity. While current methods of analysis are sufficient for the separation of achiral cannabinoid mixtures, some critical chiral pairs like cannabichromene cannot be separated fully. This is where the use of polysaccharide CSPs is and will continue to be important, as a chiral resolution will be needed to satisfy these potential requirements. This chapter will cover an introduction and evolution of polysaccharide CSPs, including a discussion on their unique separations mechanism, and review a number of the applications described in the literature of their uses for the achiral and chiral separation of cannabinoids.

Keywords: polysaccharide chiral stationary phases, cannabinoids, high-performance liquid chromatography (HPLC), super-critical fluid chromatography (SFC), chiral separations, achiral separations

1. Introduction

Polysaccharide-based chiral stationary phases (CSPs) have been reported in the literature for nearly 50 years as of the writing of this chapter. Hesse and Hagel made the first practical reports in 1973 using microcrystalline triacetylcellulose (MCTA) as a chiral separation medium, with a simple chiral model [1]. From this initial report, the applications have grown thanks to the advancements made by Prof. Yoshio Okamoto and many others, to include applications in the production of commercialized pharmaceuticals, polypeptides and biologics, natural products, and more recently, cannabis.

As a natural product, cannabis contains a wide range of compounds including, but not limited to, cannabinoids, terpenes, and other plant-based compounds [2]. These compounds typically exist as a single isomer as a requirement for further downstream processes. That is, many biological processes are enzymatically controlled, and require specific molecule confirmation for proper interaction and recognition. Therefore, biological systems have evolved to produce said single isomer that matches this confirmation. Common achiral phases like octadecylsilyl (ODS or C_{18}) and other non-polar analogs have therefore been successfully used for the separation and analysis of cannabis and cannabis-related products, as they are capable of separating achiral mixtures exclusively ([3–7] as examples). CSPs have been underutilized as a solution for the separation of such compounds and mixtures, as their cost and specialization have been seen as prohibitive or unnecessary. However, it is well established that polysaccharide CSPs are capable of performing both chiral and achiral separations, so they represent a unique opportunity for investigators to perform two types of separations at the same time. The nature of polysaccharide CSPs is unlike that of typical achiral phases. The polymeric structure of the CSPs, either cellulose or amylose-based, along with their functionalization with small molecule chiral selectors, creates an environment that can recognize the subtle structural differences that exist between enantiomers.

What exactly are enantiomers? The most effective way to envision this is to hold up one's left and right hand – the hands are mirror images of each other (excluding the minor differences in jewelry, fingernail length, cuts/bruises, etc.), but are not superimposable. When you try to overlap them, there is clearly a difference in the structure, i.e. the geometry, of the hands. Compounds that are enantiomers are the same – they have the same combination of atoms or chemical groups connected (bonded) to a single atomic center (also referred to as a stereogenic center or chiral center – usually it is carbon, but can also be nitrogen, phosphorus, or sulfur). Enantiomers differ from each other in the configuration of said atoms or chemical groups around the chiral center. They can also arise from other elements of symmetry like a plane and/or axis where two distinct confirmations can exist. An example of the latter would be atropisomers. Atropisomers contain a rotatable single bond, but because of steric hindrance (a blockage caused by large/bulky groups), are locked into two distinct confirmations. These geometric differences are not exploitable by achiral SPs, but they are by polysaccharide CSPs.

This chapter will begin with a discussion on the mechanism by which polysaccharide CSPs are capable of separating achiral and chiral analytes. This is important to understand why CSPs are so effective in their function, and why they play an important role moving forward in the separation and analysis of cannabis and cannabinoids. This will be followed by a brief sharing of established and practical examples of CSP applications in a range of mature fields (pharmaceutical and agricultural for example). The chapter will conclude with numerous examples in the literature for the separation of cannabinoids on polysaccharide-based CSPs, under various mobile phase modes including normal phase and reversed phase high performance liquid chromatography (HPLC) and supercritical fluid chromatography (SFC).

2. A brief history of polysaccharide CSPs and their separation mechanism

Traditional achiral separations on widely available phases like ODS or silica are governed primarily by polarity. That is, the difference in polarity between the analytes (compounds) and the polarity of the stationary phase (SP). With a simple enough model, one can easily predict elution order based simply on the chemical structure (or polarity) of the analyte and the polarity of the SP. As a simple example, for the separation of phenol and toluene on a C_{18} column with a mixture of acetronitrile/water, one would expect that phenol should elute first as it is more polar than toluene, which will be more strongly attracted/retained on the non-polar C_{18} SP. The same modeling cannot be performed for chiral separations however, as enantiomers are equal in their polarity. As described above in the Introduction, enantiomers differ only by the geometry in which their atoms or functional groups are arranged around the chiral center. This geometric difference can only be exploited by a medium that can create an environment that facilitates chiral recognition, which is why CSPs are a critical tool for enantiomeric separations. A well-established (yet highly unpredictable) series of intermolecular interactions helps CSPs to distinguish these subtle differences to elicit a chiral separation.

2.1 Polysaccharide chiral stationary phase separation mechanism

At the core of polysaccharide CSPs are three components: the silica gel support material, the polysaccharide backbone (either cellulose or amylose), and the chiral selector (see **Figures 1** and **2** for examples). The support material does not have too much of a role to play in the separation of enantiomers, but is important to provide CSPs with a rigidity and robustness to be used under high-pressure applications. The chiral selector and polysaccharide backbone are responsible for creating an environment that is able to distinguish the two enantiomers via a series of well-documented intermolecular (between two molecules) interactions that arise from it (see **Table 1**). When contained within in an enclosed system like a packed, chromatographic column, the potential combination of interactions is capable of producing a separation of the enantiomers. The chiral selector is key to creating these interactions - hydrogen

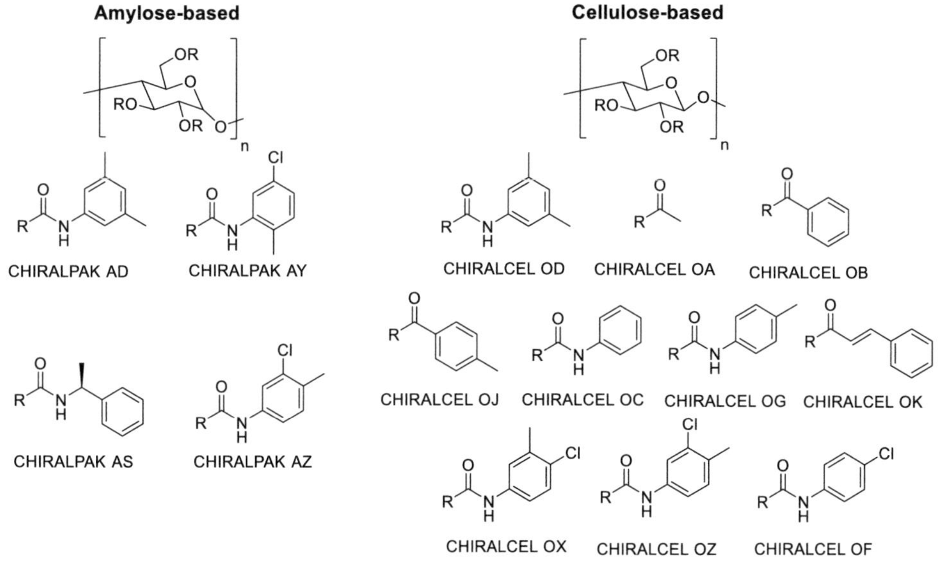

Figure 1.
Examples of structures of chiral selectors and names of coated polysaccharide-based CSPs.

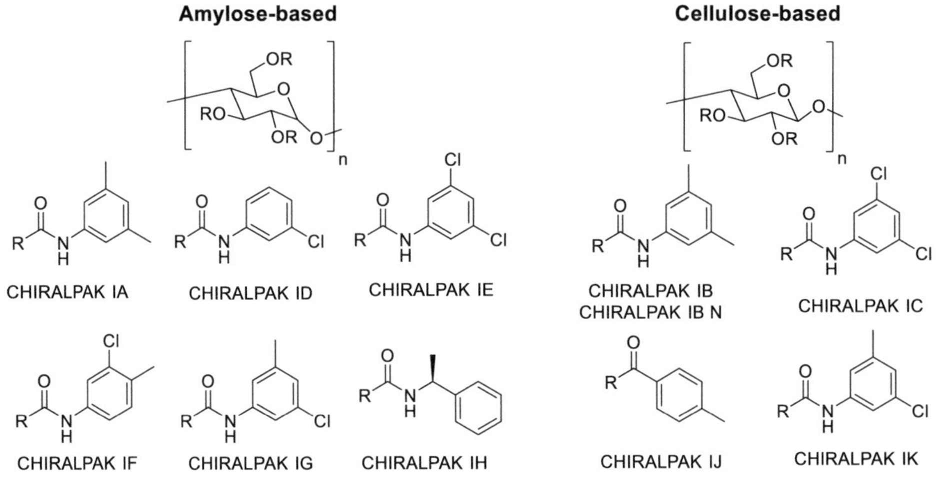

Figure 2.
Examples of structures of chiral selectors and names of immobilized polysaccharide-based CSPs.

Type of interaction	Strength	Direction	Working distance
Hydrogen bonding	Very strong	Attractive	Long range
Steric hindrance	Weak to very strong	Repulsive	Short range
π-π Interaction	Strong	Attractive	Medium range
Dipole–dipole	Intermediate	Attractive	Short range

Table 1.
Several intermolecular forces known to occur between analyte and polysaccharide CSPs. Adapted from ref. [8].

bonding, π-π stacking, dipole forces, inclusion, and repulsion can exploit the subtle differences between the enantiomer geometries [8].

Polysaccharide CSPs are unique in their ability to combine all of the above-mentioned differentiating interactions (**Table 1**) into a macromolecule that is capable of interaction with the racemic (chiral) mixture. The type and frequency of these interactions is highly dependent on several factors: (1) the type of polysaccharide backbone (e.g., cellulose or amylose), (2) the functionalization of the chiral selectors (e.g., carbamates, benzoates and their respective substituents), and (3) the combined 3D-structure created by supporting on silica. Furthermore, the solvation, swelling, or shrinking of the derivatized polymer backbone in the presence of certain solvents or additives plays an important role. Because of these factors, the interactions that take place on polysaccharide CSPs are much more unpredictable and a systematic screening becomes an essential tool for their effective application.

2.2 Development of polysaccharide CSPs for chiral separations and applications

After Hesse and Hagel published their first work using MCTA [1], the continued development of such phases lagged for more than a decade, because of structural and chromatographic inefficiencies. Professor Yoshio Okamoto in Japan made a breakthrough in 1984 by stabilizing the polysaccharide polymer (cellulose in that case), onto a solid silica gel support [9–11]. This allowed for HPLC or high pressure applications, and improved chromatographic efficiency. The first chiral selectors utilized were coated cellulose tribenzoate and coated cellulose triacetate, later commercialized by Daicel Corporation as CHIRALCEL OA and CHIRALCEL OB respectively [12–14].

In these early examples, simple models like *trans*-stilbene oxide and Troger's base were used to demonstrate the chiral recognition of the new CSPs. The number of selectors continued growing to include coated cellulose *tris*(phenylcarbamate) (CHIRALCEL OC), coated cellulose *tris*(4-chlorophenylcarbamate) (CHIRALCEL OF), coated cellulose *tris*(4-methylphenylcarbamate) (CHIRALCEL OG), and coated cellulose *tris*(3,5-dimethylphenylcarbamate) (CHIRALCEL OD) [9–11, 15–19]. The exploration and study of amylose as a polysaccharide backbone was also critical, resulting in the development of coated amylose *tris*(3,5-dimethylphenylcarbamate) (CHIRALPAK AD), coated amylose *tris*((*S*)-α-methylbenzylcarbamate) (CHIRALPAK AS), coated amylose *tris*(5-chloro-2-methylphenylcarbamate) (CHIRALPAK AY), and coated amylose *tris*(3-chloro-4-methylphenylcarbamate) (CHIRALPAK AZ) [20–22] (see **Figure 1** for full list of coated CSP selectors).

Further advancements in the production of the CSPs added robustness and increased solvent compatibility, via the incorporation of an immobilization step. This immobilization step both cross-links the polysaccharide backbone and bonds it to the silica gel surface, leading to the insolubilization of the polymer [23–32]. This resulted in a new generation of immobilized CSPs, providing access to selectors that were previously not accessible and an expanded range of compatible solvents for expanded selectivity (see **Figure 2** for full list of immobilized CSP selectors as of the time of this publication).

This diversification of selectors allowed for an expansion of selectivity that corresponded with a widening utilization in more application areas. β-blockers [33–35] and non-steroidal anti-inflammatory drugs (NSAIDs) [36–38] were two of the first classes of compounds to be screened for chiral recognition. Relevant examples included, but were not limited to, acebutolol and propranolol (β-blockers), ibuprofen and naproxen (NSAIDs). Other classes of compounds included proton-pump inhibitors like omeprazole [39–41], anti-histamines like cetirizine and meclizine [42–44], selective serotonin reuptake inhibitors (SSRIs) like sertraline and citalopram [45–47], and commercialized pharmaceuticals like Modafinil [48], Keppra [49], and Bicalutamide [50].

Agrochemicals have also become an important application area, as many pesticides, herbicides, and insecticides contain a chiral center. This application area historically received minimal attention, as there was no requirement to assess biological activity of these compounds, like there is/was for pharmaceuticals. However government regulations have changed over the last few decades, and polysaccharide CSPs have been critical for these analyses as well. There have been many papers published covering the separation of compounds like malathion, fipronil, metalaxyl, dichlorodiphenyltrichloroethane (DDT), bromuconazole, and etoxazole (as examples) [51–53]. The analysis of food has been an important application, as composition analysis is important for nutritional integrity and quality assurance. Many examples for the analysis and separation of flavanone, diketopiperizine, and naringenin-based compounds have been reported [54–56].

3. The separation of cannabinoids on polysaccharide CSPs

As mentioned in the introduction, CSPs have historically been overlooked for the analysis and separation of cannabinoids. This came primarily from the belief that cannabis did not contain any racemic pairs of compounds, or at least not any that were of particular interest. This has of course changed with the identification of cannabichromene (CBC) and cannabicyclol (CBL), as well as the rise of synthetic sources of cannabinoids, which have the potential to produce non-naturally occurring opposite enantiomers. This has also been affected by the understanding that polysaccharide CSPs are just as capable of separating achiral mixtures as they are chiral mixtures. CSPs were initially designed to exploit the subtle geometric differences that exist between enantiomers, but they are also capable of distinguishing between more pronounces achiral differences is structure.

3.1 High performance liquid chromatography (HPLC) separations

One of the earliest reports for the use of polysaccharide-based CSP for the separation of cannabinoids came from Levin *et al.* in 1993 [57]. This group used normal phase HPLC (defined as a mobile phase which contains a mixture of alkane [hexane or heptane] and alcohol [ethanol or isopropanol]), to achieve baseline resolution of several cannabinoid pairs, using CHIRALPAK AD. In 1994, Levin *et al.* published a paper using the methods developed in their original work, to explore the role of hydroxyl substitution (that is an oxygen with a hydrogen attached to it) and its effect on the chiral separation [58]. By acetylating (adding an acetyl group – carbon doubled-bonded to an oxygen, with a methyl group also attached to the carbon) the hydroxyl groups in the native cannabinoid structure, the resolution of most enantiomer pairs was decreased or lost entirely. In light of the discussion in Section 1 on the separations mechanism, this is not entirely surprising, although it is not often that a direct link between a structural feature and the chiral resolution can be made. A free hydroxyl group has a high potential for hydrogen bonding; given hydrogen bonding is one of the primary intermolecular interactions that takes place on column, the disruption of this interaction could be significant.

In 1995, Levin *et al.* continued their exploration of structural features of several cannabinoid pairs and the effects these had on their chiral separation [59]. Using CHIRALPAK AD again with normal phase HPLC, the group found some interesting results in particular with the enantiomeric pair of Δ^6 THC. The pair was well-resolved using hexane-isopropanol as a mobile phase where the elution order was determined to be (+) Δ^6 THC first followed by (−) Δ^6 THC second. The addition of 1% by volume of ethanol was sufficient to reverse the elution order. While a reversal of elution order is not entirely uncommon in chiral separations, the identification of the reversal can be important for method development. For an impurity analysis, it is preferred to have the impurity that needs to be quantified elute first. This ensures the impurity, which is often at a low level, does not elute in the tail of the major peak, thus obscuring the level of detection (LOD) or level of quantification (LOQ). For preparative applications, it is preferred to have the target enantiomer elute first, as a higher purity can be achieved while maximizing the recovery.

Jumping back briefly to 1994, Yan *et al.* published the synthesis and chiral separation of two hexahydrocannabinol derivatives on CHIRALCEL OD [60]. The cannabinoids were derived from nabilone, which is a synthetic derivative of Δ^9 THC. Much like previous reports, the separation was achieved with normal phase HPLC. In addition to the analytical method development and evaluation, the separation was also scaled to a preparative separation scale, allowing for the isolation and subsequent study of the effects of the individual cannabinoid isomers.

Thakar *et al.* published a paper in 2002, using CHIRALPAK AD and normal phase HPLC, for the separation of a pair of novel cannabinoid receptor ligands [61]. Using methods developed by Levin, the group was able to separate the two enantiomers and perform CB_1 and CB_2 receptor studies to demonstrate the effectiveness of one enantiomer over the other as a high-affinity ligand for potential therapeutic use.

Tarbox *et al.* presented a poster in 2009 at the Eastern Analytical Symposium on the separation of the isomers of Δ^8 and Δ^9 THC using again, CHIRALPAK AD [62]. The separation conditions were slightly modified from the previous reports, using instead ~96% by volume n-heptane with a mixture of methanol (~1%) and isopropanol (~3%). The significant decrease in mobile phase elution strength was required to achieve near-baseline resolution of the (+) Δ^8 and (+) Δ^9 THC isomers that eluted first and second respectively. Chiral Technologies later improved this same separation in 2018, which included the addition of the opposite (−) Δ^8 and (−) Δ^9 THC isomers [63]. In this application note, CHIRALPAK IF was used with normal phase HPLC to achieve baseline resolution of all four compounds. The elution order was determined to be (−) Δ^8 THC first, followed by (+) Δ^8 THC second, (+) Δ^9 THC third, and (−) Δ^9 THC fourth. The separation of the enantiomers of Δ^9 THC was shared in the same year (2018) using coated amylose *tris*(3,5-dimethylphenylcarbamate) with normal phase HPLC [64].

Umstead published a paper in 2021 for the separation of several cannabinoids, including cannabicyclol, cannabichromene, Δ^6, and Δ^{10} THC enantiomers [65]. There were several columns used for this work, including CHIRALPAK IB N-3, CHIRALPAK IG-3 (see **Figure 3**), CHIRALPAK IA-3, and CHIRALPAK IC-3. Normal phase HPLC was used including hexane-ethanol and hexane-isopropanol mobile phases ranging from 90–10 (v/v) to 98–2 (v/v) (see ref. [65] for full method details).

So far, only normal phase conditions have been reported, however aqueous mobile phases (containing water – also referred to as reversed-phase) have also been used for the separation of numerous cannabinoids. A particular advantage of using a reversed-phase (RP) mobile phase over normal phase is the MS compatibility, which assists in the analysis of complex cannabinoid mixtures. Onishi and Umstead published a paper in 2021 focused on the separation of a 10 cannabinoid mixture (which contained Tetrahydrocannabinolic Acid A (THCA-A), Cannabidiolic Acid (CBDA), delta-8 Tetrahydrocannabinol (Δ8-THC), Cannabidiol (CBD), (±)-Cannabichromene (CBC), Cannabinol (CBN), delta-9 Tetrahydrocannabinol (Δ9-THC), and Cannabigerol (CBG)) [66]. A particularly novel feature of this work was the use of ultra-high performance liquid chromatography (UHPLC) and Daicel Corporation's sub-2 μm immobilized polysaccharide CSPs for the separation.

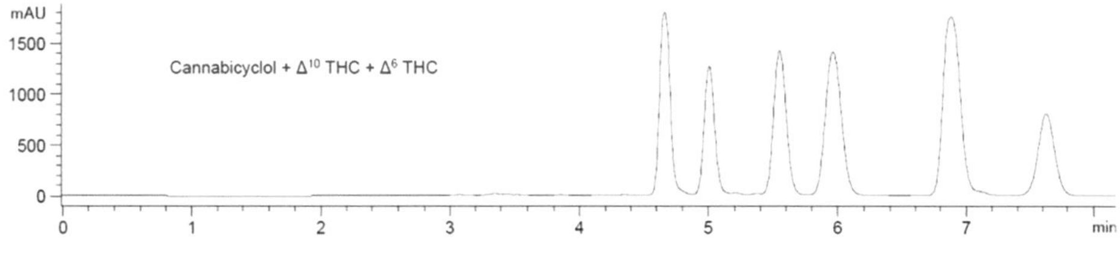

Figure 3.
Separation of cannabicyclol, Δ^6, and Δ^{10} THC under normal phase conditions of hexane-ethanol = 95–5 (v/v) on CHIRALPAK IG-3 [65].

Figure 4 shows a comparison of Van Deemter plots for the performance of 5 μm, 3 μm, and sub-2 μm CHIRALPAK IA. A Van Deemter plot is a graphical representation of three competing terms that describe the chromatographic separation of an analyte by a chromatographic column. The A term (Eddy-diffusion), B term (diffusion coefficient), and C term (resistance to mass transfer) play different roles in the overall chromatographic separation efficiency. The A term is a constant, as it is assumes the pathway length through a packed particle is more or less the same (although the actual pathway is random). The B term is also more or less constant at functional chromatographic flow rates (although it sharply decreases at very low flow, significantly less than what you would use for a separation). The C term linearly increases from zero to infinity, with the slope being less shallow for smaller particles compared to larger particles (i.e. the plate height (H) decreases much less for small particles as flow rate increases). When combined, you see curves like in **Figure 4**.

The y-axis represents the theoretical plate height (H in μm), and the x-axis linear velocity (in mm/s). Intrinsically larger particle sizes like 5 and 3 μm (in green and red respectively) have a higher theoretical plate-height due to decreased packing efficiency when packing into a column i.e. the constant A term is larger for these particle sizes. However when the linear velocity is increased, they also lose efficiency more quickly than a smaller particle (due to the C term). For this reason, faster nominal flow rates can be achieved with the smaller particles, allowing for fast/ultra-fast separations with minimal loss of resolution, or the analysis of complex samples with higher resolution.

Circling back from the short tangent on chromatographic theory, Onishi and Umstead looked at both normal phase and reversed phase HPLC, and found a number of very efficient separations. For normal phase CHIRALPAK IB-U (**Figure 5**) and CHIRALPAK IH-U were found to be the best CSPs for the separation, which used n-hexane-isopropanol-ethanol-trifluoroacetic acid = 96-3-1-0.1 (v/v) as a mobile phase.

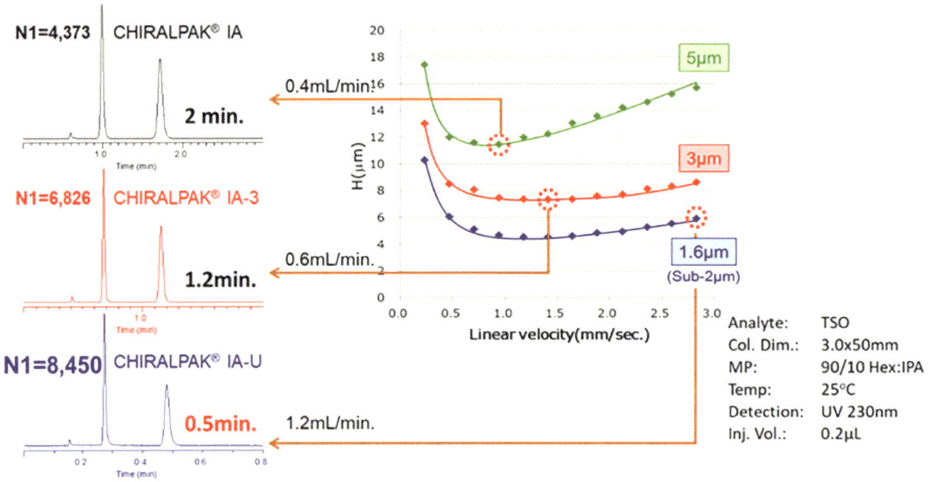

Figure 4.
Van Deemter plot for different particles sizes of CHIRALPAK IA immobilized CSP showing column efficiency related to linear velocity (flow rate) [adapted from ref. 66].

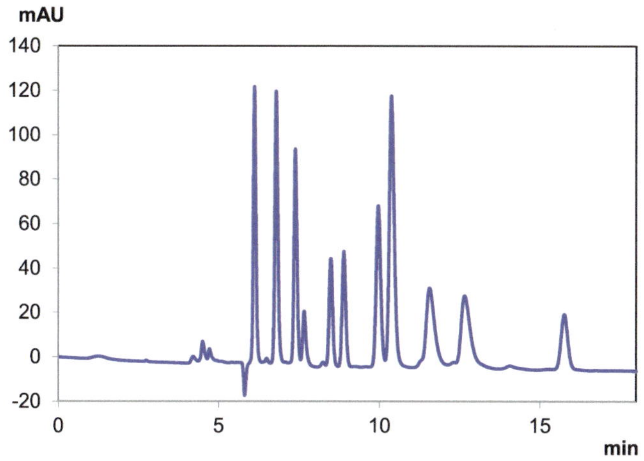

Figure 5.
10 cannabinoid mixture separation under normal phase conditions with CHIRALPAK IB-U [adapted from ref. 66].

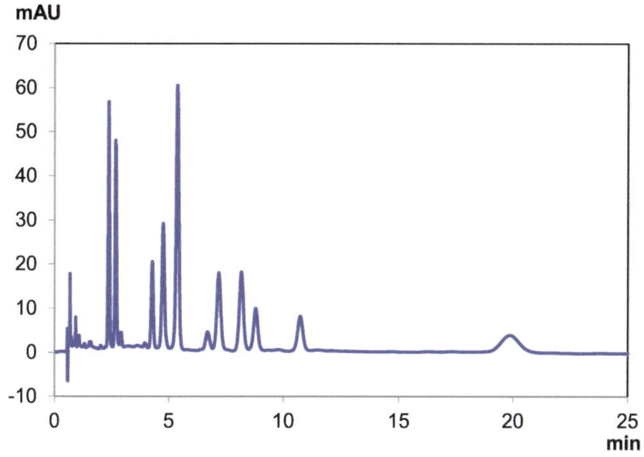

Figure 6.
10 cannabinoid mixture separation under reversed phase conditions with CHIRALPAK IG-U [adapted from ref. 66].

For reversed phase, CHIRALPAK IG-U (**Figure 6**) and CHIRALPAK ID-U were found to be the best CSPs for the separation, which utilized water/acetonitrile/trifluoroacetic acid = 45-55-0.1 (v/v) or 55-45-0.1 (v/v) respectively.

De Luca *et al.* published a paper in 2022, which covered the screening on all available immobilized-type CSPs available from Daicel Corporation (at the time of publication). They found CHIRALPAK IC and IF to be very effective at the separation of a mixture containing cannabidiolic acid (CDBA), cannabidiol (CBD), tetrahydrocannabidiolic acid (THCA), CBC (racemic), and Δ^9 THC [67]. Because CBC is a racemic cannabinoid, two peaks were observed (**Figure 7**), with good baseline resolution for all cannabinoids. The sample used for these separations was a true hemp extract (peak identification made by injection of prepared standards), so there are a number of other unidentified cannabinoids observed. For reference, the separation

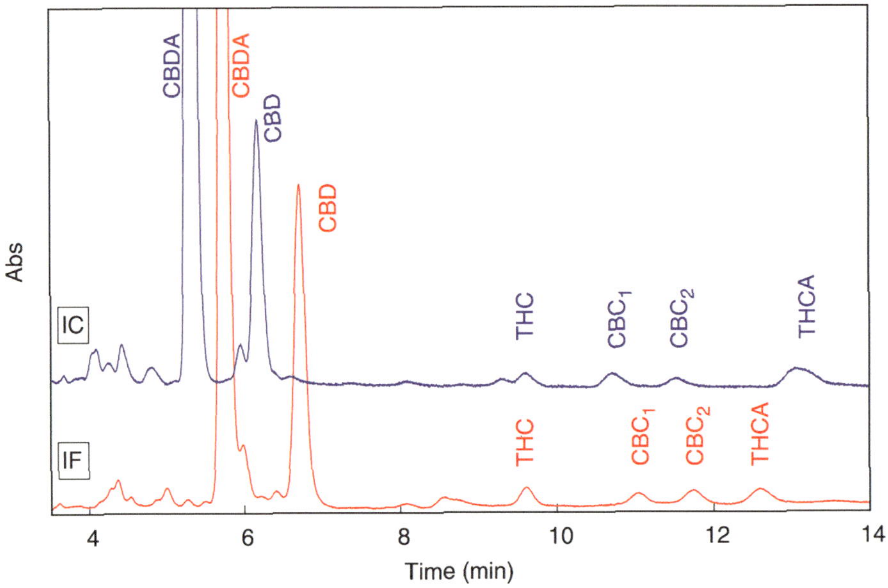

Figure 7.
Reversed phase separation of CBDA, CBD, THC, CBC, and THCA with CHIRALPAK IC (in blue) and IF (in red). Adapted from ref. [67] with author permission.

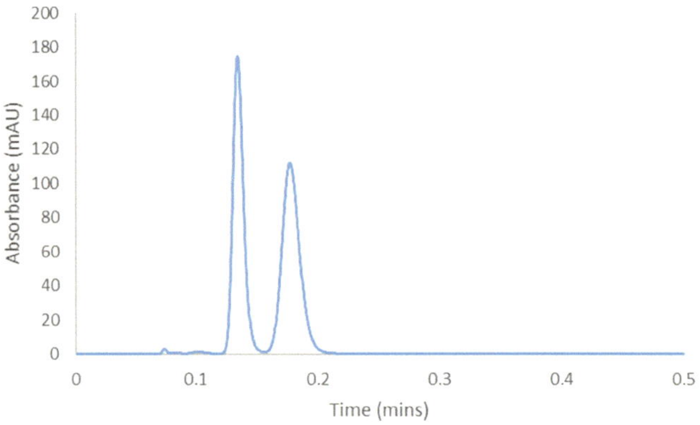

Figure 8.
Separation of (+) and (−) CBD on CHIRALPAK IG-U with Hex-EtOH = 95–5 (v/v).

in blue was achieved with isocratic elution using 60% acetonitrile and the trace in red was achieved with isocratic elution using 70% acetonitrile.

Umstead published a paper in 2022 covering the separation of CBD enantiomers under both reversed phase and normal phase HPLC [68]. For reversed phase, CHIRALPAK IA and CHIRALPAK IG were found to be the most effective CSPs for separation, using water-acetonitrile = 45–55 (v/v) or 30–70 (v/v) respectively. For normal phase HPLC, IA and IG were again found to be very effective CSPs, with the addition of CHIRALPAK ID and CHIRALPAK IE yielding good baseline resolutions as well. For the normal phase HPLC separation on IG (which used hexane-ethanol = 95–5 (v/v)), the separation was also performed on the sub-2 μm version, CHIRALPAK IG-U. This resulted in a sub-15 second separation (**Figure 8**). Similarly, the reversed phase HPLC separation on IG was repeated on IG-U, resulting in a sub-20 sec separation.

On a preparative scale, the separation of (+) and (−) Δ^9 THC was patented by Gutman *et al.* in 2016 [69]. The group used CHIRALPAK AD with methods similar to what has already been described, but rather than high-pressure application, they used a flash chromatography or medium to low pressure chromatography setup.

3.2 Super-critical fluid chromatography (SFC) separations

The mechanism for chiral separation on polysaccharide CSPs is the same for SFC as it is for HPLC, i.e., a series of intermolecular interactions between chiral analyte and chiral selector. The main difference is the composition of the mobile phase. Rather than 100% organic solvent as is the case for HPLC, SFC uses super-critical carbon dioxide (CO_2) as its primary mobile phase component. There are numerous advantages to using SFC, including the reduction of waste and associated disposal cost, overall lower viscosity mobile phases, which allows for faster flow rates i.e. faster analyses, and the ability to use methanol as a modifier, which cannot be done under normal phase HPLC (miscibility of methanol and hexane is very poor).

Toyo'oka and Kikura-Hanajiri published a paper in 2015 on the SFC separation of several synthetic cannabinoids [70]. While the work contained mostly achiral separations, there was also a reported separation of enantiomers of cis and trans cannabicyclohexanol (CCH) on coated amylose *tris*(3,5-dimethylphenylcarbamate). The separation was achieved using methanol as a modifier, and a linear gradient from 10–55% over approximately 4 mins. This was also an MS-compatible method, which assisted in peak identification of other minor cannabinoids.

Runco *et al.* published an application note on the SFC separation of Δ^8 and Δ^9 THC using coated amylose *tris*(3,5-dimethylphenylcarbamate), coated cellulose *tris*(3,5-dimethylphenylcarbamate), and coated cellulose *tris*(3-chloro-4-methylphenylcarbamate) [71]. They used ethanol as a modifier and a gradient from 2 to 20% over 5 minutes to achieve baseline resolution on all three CSPs.

Breitenbach *et al.* published a paper in 2016 covering the SFC separation of synthetic cannabinoids originating from seized drugs [72]. This group also used the three coated CSPs utilized in ref. 71, but in this instance to separate unique cannabinoid JWH-018 and its nine positional isomers. Although not fully baseline resolved, coated cellulose *tris*(3-chloro-4-methylphenylcarbamate) with isopropanol as a modifier was able to resolve eight of the 10 cannabinoids baseline.

Denicola and Barendt presented a poster in 2018 that covered the analytical separation of a series of cannabinoid mixtures ranging from 9 to 16 cannabinoids, using CHIRALPAK IB N-5 and a methanol gradient from 11 to 14% [73]. Although some partial co-elution was observed, the use of peak deconvulsion software assisted in the baseline quantification of the more complex mixtures. The method was applied to a real hemp oil sample, demonstrating the effective quantification of THC to ensure compliance with the 2018 Farm Bill requirements of less than 3% THC in CBD containing products.

Later that year, Denicola and Barendt presented a second poster that focused on the preparative separation/removal of THC from the same hemp oil sample [74]. Using the method established in the previous poster, the authors showed the isolation of 1.2 kilograms of CBD/day was possible with this new method, which at the time, was about 1.5× more productive than the achiral C18 flash chromatography method that was being used.

4. Conclusions

Polysaccharide CSPs have a rich and storied history for the separation and analysis of chiral pharmaceuticals and agrochemicals, as well as important applications in the food and cosmetic industries. Although not traditionally used for achiral separations, their unique separations mechanism allows for the exploitation of small differences in energy and molecular geometry, meaning a broader range of applicability when compared to achiral SPs. As this awareness has grown, the applications in the field of cannabis separation and analysis have grown with it, particularly over the last decade. Their ability to separate diastereomers, structural isomers, and other positional isomers present in cannabis make them well suited for these applications.

As demonstrated in the chapter their ability to be used in a wide range of mobile phases makes them suitable for numerous applications, ranging from analytical and preparative scale, and with great flexibility in detection technique (mass-assisted or ultra-violet detection for instance). No doubt as the library of natural and synthetic cannabinoids continues to grow, the need for enantiomeric resolution will grow with it. As all application areas continue to expand, particularly for medicinal use, polysaccharide-based CSPs are and will be well suited to meet the needs for chiral purity testing.

Conflict of interest

The author declare no conflict of interest.

Author details

Weston J. Umstead
Daicel Chiral Technologies, West Chester, PA, USA

*Address all correspondence to: wumstead@cti.daicel.com

References

[1] Hesse G, Hagel R. Eine vollständige Recemattennung durch eluitons-chromagographie an cellulose-tri-acetat. Chromatographia. 1973;**6**(6):277

[2] Hanuš LO, Meyer SM, Muñoz E, et al. Phytocannabinoids: A unified critical inventory. Natural Product Reports. 2016;**33**(12):1357-1392

[3] Zivovinovic S, Alder R, Allenspach MD, Steuer C. Determination of cannabinoids in *Cannabis sativa* L. samples for recreational, medical, and forensic purposes by reversed-phase liquid chromatography-ultraviolet detection. Journal of Analytical Science and Technology. 2018;**9**(27):1-10

[4] Aubin AJ, Layton C, Helmueller S. Separation of 16 Cannabinoids in Cannabis Flowers and Extracts using Reversed-Phase Isocratic HPLC Method. Massachusetts, USA: Waters Corporation Application Note; 2018

[5] Mandrioli M, Tura M, Scotti S, Gallina Toschi T. Fast detection of 10 cannabinoids by RP-HPLC-UV method in *Cannabis sativa* L. Molecules. 2019;**24**(2113):1-12

[6] Saingam W, Sakunpak A. Development and validation of reverse phase high performance liquid chromatography method for the determination of delta-9-tetrahydrocannabinol and cannabidiol in oromucosal spray from cannabis extract. Revista Brasileira de Farmacognosia. 2018;**28**(6):669-672

[7] Patel B, Wene D, Fan Z. Qualitative and quantitative measurement of cannabinoids in cannabis using modified HPLC/DAD method. Journal of Pharmaceutical and Biomedical Analysis. 2017;**146**:15-23

[8] Berthod A, editor. Chiral Recognition in Separation Methods. Berlin Heidelberg: Springer-Verlag; 2010

[9] Okamoto Y, Kawashima M, Yamamoto K, Hatada K. Useful chiral packing materials for high-performance liquid chromatographic resolution. Cellulose triacetate and tribenzoate coated on macroporous silica gel. Chemistry Letters. 1984;**13**(5):739

[10] Okamoto Y, Kawashima M, Hatada K. Chromatographic resolution. 7. Useful chiral packing materials for high-performance liquid chromatographic resolution of enantiomers: Phenylcarbamates of polysaccharides coated on silica gel. Journal of American Chemical Society. 1984;(18):106, 5357

[11] Ichida A, Shibata T, Okamoto I, Yuki Y, Namikoshi H, Toda Y. Resolution of enantiomers by HPLC on cellulose derivatives. Chromatographia. 1984;**19**:280

[12] Rimbock K, Kastner A, Mannschreck A. Microcrystalline tribenzoylcellulose: A high-performanc liquid chromatographic sorbent for the separation of enantiomers. Journal of Chromatography. 1986;**351**:346

[13] Francotte E, Wolf RM. Benzoyl cellulose beads in the pure polymeric form as a new powerful sorbent for the chromatographic resolution of racemates. Chirality. 1991;**3**(1):43

[14] Francotte E, Wolf RM. Chromatographic resolution on methylbenzoylcellulose beads: Modulation of the chiral recognition

by variation of the position of the methyl group on the aromatic ring. Journal of Chromatography. 1992;**595**(1-2):63

[15] Yashima E, Okamoto Y. Chiral discrimination on polysaccharides derivatives. Bulletin of the Chemical Society of Japan. 1995;**68**(12):91

[16] Yashima E, Yamamoto C, Okamoto Y. Polysaccharide-based chiral LC columns. Synlett. 1998;**1998**(4):344

[17] Okamoto Y, Yashima E. Polysaccharide derivatives for chromatographic separation of enantiomers. Angewandte Chemie International Edition. 1998;**37**(8):1021

[18] Okamoto Y, Aburatani R, Hatada K. Chromatographic chiral resolution: XIV. Cellulose tribenzoate derivatives as chiral stationary phases for high-performance liquid chromatography. Journal of Chromatography. 1987;**389**:95

[19] Okamoto Y, Kawashima M, Hatada K. Chromatographic resolution: XI. Controlled chiral recognition of cellulose triphenylcarbamate derivatives supported on silica gel. Journal of Chromatography A. 1986;**363**(2):173-186

[20] Okamoto Y, Aburatani R, Fukumoto T, Hatada K. Useful chiral stationary phases for HPLC. Amylose tris (3, 5-dimethylphenylcarbamate) and tris (3, 5-dichlorophenylcarbamate) supported on silica gel. Chemistry Letters. 1987;**16**(9):1857

[21] Okamoto Y, Cao Z-K, Aburatani R, Hatada K. Optical resolution of alcohols as carbamates by HPLC on cellulose tris (phenylcarbamate) derivatives. Bulletin of the Chemical Society of Japan. 1987;**60**(11):3999

[22] Okamoto Y, Aburantani R, Kaida Y, Hatada K. Direct optical resolution of carboxylic acids by chiral HPLC on tris (3, 5-dimethylphenylcarbamate) of cellulose and amylose. Chemistry Letters. 1988;**17**(7):1125

[23] Okamoto Y, Aburatani R, Miura S, Hatada K. Chiral stationary phases for HPLC: Cellulose Tris (3, 5-dimethylphenylcarbamate) and Tris (3, 5-dichlorophenylcarbamate) chemically bonded to silica gel. Journal of Liquid Chromatography. 1987;**10**:1613

[24] Yashima E, Fukaya H, Okamoto Y. 3,5-Dimethylphenylcarbamatesofcellulose and amylose regioselectively bonded to silica gel as chiral stationary phases for high-performance liquid chr. Journal of Chromatography A. 1994;**677**:11

[25] Enomoto N, Furukawa S, Osagawara Y, Akano H, Kawamura Y, Yashima E, et al. Preparation of silica gel-bonded amylose through enzyme-catalyzed polymerization and chiral recognition ability of its phenylcarbamate derivative in HPLC. Analytical Chemistry. 1996;**68**(17):2798

[26] Francotte E. Photochemically cross-linked polysaccharide derivatives as supports for the chromatographic separation of enantiomers. PCT WO 96/27615. 1996:1-32

[27] Francotte E, Huynh D. Immobilization of 3, 5-dimethylphenyl carbamate of cellulose and amylose on silica by photochemical and thermal radical processes. Chirality. 2022;**34**(5):711-731. DOI: 10.1002/chir.23426

[28] Oliveros L, Lopez P, Minguillon C, Franco P. Chiral chromatographic discrimination ability of a cellulose 3,5-dimethylphenylcarbamate/10-undecenoate mixed derivative fixed on several chromatographic matrices. Journal of Liquid Chromatography. 1995;**18**(1-2):1521

[29] Minguillon C, Franco P, Oliveros L, Lopez P. Bonded cellulose-derived high-performance liquid chromatography chiral stationary phases I. Influence of the degree of fixation on selectivity. Journal of Chromatography A. 1996; (1-2):728, 407

[30] Garces J, Franco P, Oliveros L, Minguillon C. Mixed cellulose-derived benzoates bonded on allylsilica gel as HPLC chiral stationary phases: Influence of the introduction of an aromatic moiety in the fixation substituent. Tetrahedron: Asymmetry. 2003;**14**(9):1179-1185

[31] Chen XM, Yamamoto C, Okamoto Y. Influence of vinyl monomers and temperature on immobilization of cellulose 3,5-dimethylphenylcarbamate onto silica gel as chiral stationary phases for high-performance liquid chromatography. Journal of Chromatography A. 2006;**1104**(1-2):62-68

[32] Chen XM, Liu Y, Kong I, Zou H. Synthesis of covalently bonded cellulose derivative chiral stationary phases with a bifunctional reagent of 3-(triethoxysilyl) propyl isocyanate. Journal of Chromatography A. 2003;**1010**:185

[33] Pandya PA, Shah PA, Shrivastav PS. Simultaneous enantioseparation and simulation studies of atenolol, metoprolol and propranolol on Chiralpak® IG column using supercritical fluid chromatography. Journal of Pharmaceutical Analysis. 2021;**11**:746-756

[34] Garzotti M, Hamdan M. Supercritical fluid chromatography coupled to electrospray mass spectrometry: A powerful tool for the analysis of chiral mixtures. Journal of Chromatography B. 2002;**770**(1-2):53-61

[35] Maftouh M, Granier-Loyaux C, Chavana E, Marini J, Pradines A, Vander Heydan Y, et al. Screening approach for chiral separation of pharmaceuticals: Part III. Supercritical fluid chromatography for analysis and purification in drug discovery. Journal of Chromatography A. 2005;**1088**(1-2):67-81

[36] Zhang T, Nguyen N, Franco P, Vollmer M. Separation of Enantiomers and Conformers of Tofisopam. Santa Clara, California, USA: Agilent Application Note; 2011. Available from: http://www.chem.agilent.com/Library/applications/5990-9315EN.pdf

[37] Lee J, Lee JT, Watts WL, Barendt J, Yan TQ, Huang Y, et al. On the method development of immobilized polysaccharide chiral stationary phases in supercritical fluid chromatography using an extended range of modifiers. Journal of Chromatography A. 2014;**1374**:238-246

[38] Okamoto Y, Aburatani R, Kaida Y, Hatada K, Inotsume N, Nakano M. Direct chromatographic separation of 2-arylpropionic acid enantiomers using tris(3,5-dimethylphenylcarbamate)s of cellulose and amylose as chiral stationary phases. Chirality. 1989;**1**(3):239-242

[39] Chennuru LN, Choppari T, Duvvuri S, Dubey PK. Enantiomeric separation of proton pump inhibitors on new generation chiral columns using LC and supercritical fluid chromatography. Journal of Separation Science. 2013;**36**(18):3004-3010

[40] Rahman A, Haque MR, Sultan Z, Rahmna MM, Rashid MA. Enantiomeric determination of omeprazole and esomeprazole by a developed and validated chiral HPLC method and stability studies by microthermal analysis. Journal of Pharmaceutical Sciences. 2017;**16**:221-233

[41] Cirilli R, Ferretti R, Gallinella B, Turchetto L, Zanitti L, La Torre F. Development and validation of

an enantioselective and chemoselective HPLC method using a Chiralpak IA column to simultaneously quantify (R)-(+)- and (S)-(−)-lansoprazole enantiomers and related impurities. Journal of Pharmaceutical and Biomedical Analysis. 2009;**50**(1):9-14

[42] Eom HY, Kang M, Kang SW, Kim U, Suh JH, Kim J, et al. Rapid chiral separation of racemic cetirizine in human plasma using subcritical fluid chromatography-tandem mass spectrometry. Journal of Pharmaceutical and Biomedical Analysis. 2016;**117**:380-389

[43] Liu Q, Zhang Z, Bo H, Sheldon RA. Direct separation of the enantiomers of cetirizine and related compounds by reversed-phase chiral HPLC. Chromatographia. 2002;**56**:233-235

[44] Liu Y, Wang X, Yu J, Guo X. Chiral separation and molecular simulation study of six antihistamine agents on a coated cellulose tri-(3,5-dimethylphenycarbamate) column (Chiralcel OD-RH) and its recognition mechanisms. Electrophoresis. 2021;**42**:1461-1472

[45] Rosetti A, Ferretti R, Zanitti L, Casulli A, Villani C, Cirilli R. Single-run reversed-phase HPLC method for determining sertraline content, enantiomeric purity, and related substances in drug substance and finished product. Journal of Pharmaceutical Analysis. 2020;**10**:610-616

[46] Jiang C-J, Chen Z-R, Zeng H. Chiral separation of sertraline hydrochloride by HPLC. Chinese Journal of Pharmaceutical Analysis. 2007;**27**(7):997-998

[47] Umstead WJ. The Chiral Resolution of Fluoxetine. Chiral Technologies Application Note; 2022

[48] Hauck W, Adam P, Bobier C, Landmesser N. Use of large-scale chromatography in the preparation of armodafinil. Chirality. 2008;**20**(8): 896-899

[49] Futagawa T, Canvat JP, Deleers M, Hamende M, Zimmermann V. Process for the preparation of levetiracetam. US Patent US 6,107-492. 2000

[50] Sadutto D, Ferretti R, Zanitti L, Casulli A, Cirilli R. Analytical and semipreparative high performance liquid chromatography enantioseparation of bicalutamide and its chiral impurities on an immobilized polysaccharide-based chiral stationary phase. Journal of Chromatography A. 2016;**1445**:166-171

[51] Paolini L, Hausser N, Zhang T. Chiral resolution of the insecticide fipronil enantiomers and the simultaneous determination of its major transformation products by high-performance liquid chromatography interfaced with mass spectrometry. Chirality. 2022;**34**:473-483

[52] Ellington J, Evans JJ, Prickett KB, Champion WL. High-performance liquid chromatographic separation of the enantiomers of organophosphorus pesticides on polysaccharide chiral stationary phases. Journal of Chromatography A. 2001;**928**(2):145-154

[53] Champion WL Jr, Watts WL Jr, Umstead WJ. The separation of several organophosphate pesticides on immobilized polysaccharide chiral stationary phases. In: Chirality, Early View. 2022

[54] Schaffrath M, Weidmann V, Maison W. Enantioselective high performance liquid chromatography and supercritical fluid chromatography separation of spirocyclic terpenoid flavor compounds. Journal of Chromatography A. 2014;**1363**:270-277

[55] Martinez SE, Davies NM. Stereospecific quantitation of 6-prenylnaringenin in commercially available H. lupulus-containing natural health products and dietary supplements. Research in Pharmaceutical Sciences. 2015;**10**(3):182-191

[56] Qiao X, An R, Huang Y, Li S, Li L, Tzeng YM, et al. Separation of 25R/S-ergostane triterpenoids in the medicinal mushroom Antrodia camphorata using analytical supercritical-fluid chromatography. Journal of Chromatography A. 2014;**1358**:252-260

[57] Levin S, Abu-Lafi S, Zahalka J, Mechoulam R. Resolution of chiral cannabinoids on amylose tris(3,5-dimethylphenylcarbamate) chiral stationary phase: Effects of structural features and mobile phase additive. Journal of Chromatography A. 1993;**654**(1):53-64

[58] Abu-Lafi S, Sterin M, Levin S. Role of hydroxyl groups in chiral recognition of cannabinoids by carbamated amylose. Journal of Chromatography A. 1994;**679**(1):47-58

[59] Levin S, Sterin S, Abu-Lafi S. Structural features affecting chiral resolution of cannabimimetic enantiomers by amylose 3,5-dimethylphenylcarbamate chiral stationary phase. Chirality. 1995;7(3):140-146

[60] Yan G, Yin D, Khanolkar AD, Compton DR, Martin BR, Makriyannis A. Synthesis and pharmacological properties of 11-hydroxy-3-(1′,1′-dimethylheptyl) hexahydrocannabinol: A high affinity cannabinoid agonist. Journal of Medicinal Chemistry. 1994;**37**(16):2619-2622

[61] Thakur GA, Palmer SL, Harrington PE, Stergiades IA, Tius MA, Makriyannis M. Enantiomeric resolution of a novel chiral cannabinoid receptor ligand. Journal of Biochemical and Biophysical Methods. 2002;**54**(1-3): 415-422

[62] Tarbox T, Dilek I, Sreenivasen U, Yaser K. A Validated Chiral HPLC Method for Resolution of Δ8 and Δ9 - Tetrahydrocannabinol Enantiomers T. Tarbox, Poster Presented at EAS, Cerilliant Corporation; 2009

[63] Chiral Technologies. Application Note – Separation of the Enantiomers of (+/−) Δ8-THC and (+/−) Δ9-THC. West Chester, Pennsylvania, USA: Chiral Technologies; 2018

[64] YMC Europe GmbH. Application Note – Fast and Easy Achiral & Chiral Analysis of Cannabinoids. 2018

[65] Umstead WJ. The separation of several minor cannabinoids via chiral HPLC. Cannabis Science and Technology. 2021;**4**(6):44-51

[66] Onishi T, Umstead WJ. The separation of cannabinoids on Sub-2 μm immobilized polysaccharide chiral stationary phases. Pharmaceuticals. 2021;**14**(12):1250

[67] De Luca C, Buratti A, Umstead W, Franco P, Cavazzini A, Felletti S, et al. Investigation of retention behavior of natural cannabinoids on differently substituted polysaccharide-based chiral stationary phases under reversed-phase liquid chromatographic conditions. Journal of Chromatography A. 2022;**1672**:463076-463084

[68] Umstead WJ. The chiral separation of the (+) and (−) enantiomers of cannabidiol (CBD). Cannabis Science and Technology. 2022;**5**(5):30-37

[69] Gutman AL, Etinger M, Fedotev I, Khanolkar R, Nisnevich GA, Pertsikov B et al. Methods for Purifying

trans-(−)-Δ9-Tetrahydrocannabinol and Trans-(+)-Δ9-Tetrahydrocannabinol, US Patent 9,278,083 B2. 2016

[70] Toyo'oka T, Kikura-Hanajiri R. A reliable method for the separation and detection of synthetic cannabinoids by supercritical fluid chromatography with mass spectrometry, and its application to plant products. Chemical and Pharmaceutical Bulletin. 2015;**63**(10):762-769

[71] Runco J, Aubin A, Layton C. The Separation of Δ8-THC, Δ9-THC, and their Enantiomers by UPC2 using Trefoil Chiral Columns. Application Note, Waters Corporation; 2016

[72] Breitenbach S, Rowe WF, McCord B, Lurie IS. Assessment of ultra high performance supercritical fluid chromatography as a separation technique for the analysis of seized drugs: Applicability to synthetic cannabinoids. Journal of Chromatography A. 2016;**1440**(1):201-211

[73] Denicola C, Barendt J. Streamlined Cannabinoid and Potency Assays Utilizing HPLC and SFC. Cannabis Sciences Conference Poster. West Chester, Pennsylvania, USA: Chiral Technologies; 2018

[74] Denicola C, Barendt J. Cannabinoid Isolation Models Utilizing Immobilized Chiral Stationary Phases and SFC. Emerald Conference Poster. West Chester, Pennsylvania, USA: Chiral Technologies; 2018

Chapter 2

Cannabis Medicines: Guidance for the Selection, Purchase and Supply for Clinical Trials

Peter Galettis, John Barlow, Jaroslav Boublik, Stefania Capra, Rachel Galettis, Myfanwy Graham, Courtney Hill, Paul Mavor, Jasminka Nikolajevic-Sarunac, Rosemary Richards, Janet Schloss, Melinda Thompson, Linda Truong, Berzenn Urbi, Katrina Weston-Green and Aaron K. Wong

Abstract

Cannabis medicines are in demand from the public for treating a range of diseases and symptoms; however, clinicians are reluctant to prescribe these products because of limited evidence and prescribing information. To generate this evidence, quality clinical trials of cannabis medicines must be undertaken, yet their design is a complex, often uncharted territory, and involves the cooperation and sharing of knowledge of multiple stakeholders. Before designing a clinical trial, researchers require a clear understanding of the potential therapeutic benefit cannabis medicines may have, the form and formulation of the product, and the dose to be investigated. Researchers must also be aware of the applicable pharmaceutical regulations in the country or jurisdiction where the research is to be undertaken, as well as manufacturing or licensing regulations that may be imposed at the source of the cannabis product. Importantly, collaborations with industry are a key to the successful outcome of cannabis medicines clinical trials. Without funding and sponsorship of clinical trials, the ability to generate quality data will be limited and the evidence for cannabis medicines to be registered as therapeutics lacking. Collaborations between researchers, industry, and regulators, working together in sharing knowledge, are therefore critical to generate high quality cannabis medicines research.

Keywords: cannabis medicines, product selection, clinical Trials, drug-drug interactions, dosage forms

1. Introduction

Since the Federal legalization of cannabis medicines in Australia in 2016, cannabis has rapidly moved from being a recreational drug to a medicinal product. While it shows great therapeutic promise, one of the issues faced by clinicians in prescribing cannabis is the limited information available from high quality clinical trials across a broad range of indications. In order to generate this evidence, collaboration and sharing of knowledge between all stakeholders will be required to progress quality clinical trials of cannabis medicines. This paper discusses several issues that investigators have found when designing clinical studies using cannabis medicines as investigational products. These include cannabis medicine selection according to the indication(s) being studied, dosage form, dose range, drug-drug interactions, regulatory considerations, purchase and supply, purity and consistency of plant-based products, and industry engagement.

2. Selection of cannabis medicines for indications

Over 120 phytocannabinoids have been identified in Cannabis sativa L. that have a diverse range of molecular targets [1]. Consideration of the type of cannabinoid and its pharmacokinetics and pharmacodynamics is important when selecting products for clinical trials [2]. To date, research has focused heavily on cannabidiol (CBD) and Δ-9-tetrahydrocannabinol (THC). Cannabis medicine clinical trials can be located on clinical trial registries, such as the Australian New Zealand Clinical Trials Registry (ANZCTR), ClinicalTrials.gov and WHO International Clinical Trials Registry Platform (ICTRP) [3–5]. The selection of cannabis medicines for a particular indication in the context of a clinical trial requires researchers to consider several different factors.

Some trials have investigated a combination of cannabinoids. For example, in palliative care [6] and glioblastoma [7], THC and CBD have been trialed in the ratios of 1:1 and 4:1, respectively. Trials of CBD alone have been conducted in anxiety and schizophrenia [8] and refractory epilepsy (Dravet syndrome and Lennox-Gastaut syndrome) [9]. Nabiximols, an oral spray containing roughly equal parts CBD and THC and marketed under the trade name Sativex, has been studied in spasticity in multiple sclerosis [10], cannabis dependence [11], and neuropathic pain [12]. Dronabinol, an entirely synthetic form of THC has been trialed for anorexia and weight loss in patients with acquired immune deficiency syndrome [13] while dronabinol and nabilone, also a synthetic cannabinoid that is similar to THC but appears to be more potent, have both been studied in treatment-refractory chemotherapy-induced nausea and vomiting [14]. Dementia studies have trialed THC, dronabinol, and nabilone [15].

These are only a few examples of numerous trials for different clinical indications and disease states. Many of these studies have had mixed results suggesting that proposed clinical trials, especially for diseases not already studied will require a thorough examination of in vitro and preclinical work to inform the selection of the cannabinoid formulation most appropriate for the disease under study.

To this end, there is an abundance of in vitro and in vivo studies being conducted on a variety of cannabinoids and in different formulations that over time, will help identify the principal components required of a cannabinoid for the disease being targeted [1]. As always, a detailed literature search is essential.

3. Selection of the form of cannabis medicines

Several factors need to be considered when selecting a cannabis medicine for use in a clinical trial. Key features include the age of the patient cohort where participants may have limited dexterity in handling certain formulations, likely comorbid conditions that may affect drug absorption, and manufacturers' ability to create a placebo that looks, tastes, and smells the same as the investigational product.

Several different dosage formulations can be selected. **Table 1** describes the potential advantages and disadvantages of common dosage forms of cannabis medicines that may be considered for use in a clinical trial. Less common dosage forms such as rectal, vaginal, and intravenous are not discussed as they are generally less practical forms for a clinical trial in comparison with the forms discussed below [16].

4. Dose selection

Currently, dosing information is only available for approved cannabis medicines, dronabinol, nabilone, nabiximols and Epidiolex (CBD). For unregistered cannabis medicines, there is no precise dosing recommendation. Pharmacokinetic variability of cannabinoids is very high both among and between cohorts and hence, dosing is highly individualized and dependant on the patient's condition [21, 22]. Generally, the approach for cannabis dosing is to start low and go slow. The patient should be started on a low dose and gradually titrated until a therapeutic effect without any undesired side effect is achieved [23–26].

Most patients take oral cannabis medicines 2–3 times per day. Epidiolex, a cannabis-derived form of CBD, is taken twice daily with a starting dose of 5 mg/kg/day up to a maximum dose of 20 mg/kg/day [27], while nabiximols is taken as 4 to 8 sprays/day (1 spray is equivalent to 2.7 mg THC and 2.5 mg CBD) up to a maximum of 12 sprays/day [28]. Frequency is dependent on the duration of action, which is in the order of 3–4 hours for inhaled products and 8–12 hours for oral products.

THC-dominant products can be taken at bedtime for days 1–2 to minimize undesirable daytime side effects such as dizziness or drowsiness and encourage tolerance of doses beginning at 2.5 mg of THC. If the dose is tolerated, the dosing can be doubled every 1–2 days until any undesired side effect(s) are experienced. In this event, patients are advised to revert to their previous dose [23].

CBD dominant products can be used at higher concentrations than THC products because they produce fewer adverse effects. Doses of CBD between 1 and 50 mg/kg/day improve psychotic symptoms, seizures, and anxiety [29]. An average CBD dose of 15 mg/kg/day showed positive significant reductions of seizure while CBD between 150 and 600 mg/day produced therapeutic effects in social anxiety disorder and insomnia. The maximum tolerated dose for CBD in humans is 1500 mg/day [30]. This data shows that CBD-dominant products have a higher therapeutic index than THC-dominant products. Patients are advised to keep a journal of their cannabis medicine dosing together with a record of their symptoms to aid in determining the optimal CBD dose for their particular condition.

5. Drug-drug interactions

There is variable evidence indicating other drugs interact with cannabis medicines, ranging from hypothetical concepts to documented clinical trial evidence [31, 32]. Interactions among drugs is particularly relevant in trials where a variety of pharmacologic products is being investigated. Drug-drug interactions may increase

Route of delivery	Dosage Form	Advantages	Disadvantages
Inhaled	Smoked or vaporized	• Rapid onset peak plasma concentrations 3–10 minutes) [2] • Higher bioavailability (10–35%) [2, 17] • May be suitable for those with difficulty administering other formulations • Bypasses first pass metabolism [16]	• Difficult to determine the total amount of product inhaled or absorbed, leading to unintended bias • Difficult to reliably titrate dose when dose inhaled is uncertain [16] • May be less portable depending on device used to vaporize product • Bystanders exposed to inhaled product • Matched placebo comparatively challenging to formulate • Smell of the product is noticeable
Sublingual	Sprays, oils, tinctures, wafer	• Rapid onset • Higher bioavailability • Liquid version amendable to fine titration • Suitable for patients with swallowing difficulties • Bypasses first metabolism [16]	• Alcohol-based products may cause pain in participants with mucositis • Participants may not be able to reliably hold sublingual product under tongue for an adequate duration • Bottles and syringes required are challenging for the elderly who may have poor eyesight or arthritis • Difficult to formulate an identical placebo • Potential for spillage of liquid product • Taste of product is noticeable • Best absorption after meals [18]
Oral	Capsules, tablets, oils, tinctures	• Easiest to create matched placebo • Capsule or tablet version have minimal issues with taste • Liquid version amenable to fine titration by volume • Acid resistant coating for encapsulated product can avoid gastric degradation • Can be packed into blister packs to aid administration for those with dexterity issues • Measurable quantity is consumed reducing confounding from inadequate consumption	• Slower onset of action [16, 19] • Longer duration to peak plasma concentration (120 minutes) [2, 16, 19] • Lower bioavailability [16, 19] • Undergoes first-pass metabolism [16] • Not suitable with gastrointestinal absorption issues (e.g. colitis, intestinal obstruction) or difficulty swallowing • Packaging in tamper-proof bottles may cause difficulty for the elderly who may have dexterity issues • Bottles and syringes required are challenging for those with poor eyesight or arthritis • Potential for spillage of liquid product • Taste of liquid product is noticeable

Route of delivery	Dosage Form	Advantages	Disadvantages
Topical	Creams, patches	• Higher bioavailability [16] • Steady dose delivery over a prolonged time period [16] • Easy to administer [16] • May be helpful for local symptoms (e.g. pain) • Comparatively less challenging to create a matching placebo • Suitable for most patients as comorbid conditions are less likely to affect absorption • Bypasses first-pass metabolism [16, 20]	• Possible skin reaction to drug or adhesive • Patches may prematurely burst open • Need for education on correct techniques of application (e.g. site rotation, avoiding unsuitable sites) • Not suitable for participants with widespread skin conditions

Table 1.
Advantages and disadvantages of common dosage forms of Cannabis medicines when used in a clinical trial setting.

the active concentration of cannabinoids, enhancing the possibility of adverse effects, or they may decrease cannabinoid concentrations, compromising their physiologic effects [33]. The converse effect might be expected from the competing drug.

Examples of drug-drug interactions include blood pressure-lowering medications, warfarin [33], antiepileptic drugs (e.g. clobazam) [34], and central nervous system depressant medications, including opioids and benzodiazepines [35]. Researchers should keep in mind that drug-drug interactions can occur with cannabis medicines.

6. Regulatory, purchase and supply

Clinical trials place stringent demands upon the availability of precise and reproducible formulations of the medicines under study. Unfortunately, the quality and consistency of supply of many cannabis medicines are not of a standard that would facilitate their use in most clinical trials. Indeed, while plant genetics can be tightly regulated through cloning techniques to minimize variability amongst cannabis plants, multiple factors can still alter the phytochemical profile of plant-based medicines, including environmental factors, time of harvest, manufacturing processes and storage conditions (reviewed in [36]). In Australia, to overcome this the Therapeutic Goods Administration (TGA) has introduced guidelines for cannabis medicines and more recently the U.S. Food and Drug Administration (FDA) has also introduced guidelines [37, 38]. Cannabis medicines used in clinical trials must align with the existing framework for the use of medications in clinical trials, and meet the requirements for human use of cannabis medicines set by the local regulator e.g. FDA, European Medicines Agency (EMA), TGA [39–41]. Local pharmaceutical, prescribing and holding regulations, approvals, and requirements for labelling, transport, and storage of investigational medicinal product for use in a clinical trial must also be confirmed prior to selecting and purchasing a product for a clinical trial [42–44].

Australia's TGA approves the use of medicines in a clinical trial through their Clinical Trial Notification (CTN) scheme [41, 45]. Prescribed cannabis medicines must conform to Therapeutic Goods Orders No. 93 (Standard for Medicinal Cannabis) (TGO 93) and TGO 100 (Microbiological quality of medicinal cannabis products), among others [37, 46, 47]. Adherence to Good Manufacturing Process (GMP), and to federal and state pharmacy regulations, policies, and their respective drugs and poisons legislation is required [48–52]. Where the manufacture of cannabis medicine products will form part of a clinical trial, a license authorising manufacture for clinical trial use must be in place between the manufacturer and the TGA [44, 53].

Following product feasibility, risk review, and final selection, supply contracts should be developed for the purchase of the product(s) for the clinical trial, to document agreed requirements, roles, and responsibilities including:

- Formulation (dose, volume, and form)

- Packaging and labeling requirements (if required) must comply with Pharmaceutical Inspection Convention and Pharmaceutical Inspection Co-operative Scheme (PIC/S) Annex 13 [43, 44]

- Consistency of supply (i.e. volume, consistency and purity of product supplied across the duration of the clinical trial) with an agreement to provide certificates of analysis with each batch to ensure purity and consistency in phytochemical profile

- Availability of stock

- Cost

- Any regulatory fees, import permits as required, shipping costs

- Insurance and indemnity

- Access to data if appropriate (this may be an ethics committee decision)

- Pharmacovigilance reporting responsibilities

- Confirmation that all products under trial will meet and be maintained in compliance with International Conference for Harmonisation of technical requirements for pharmaceuticals for human use Good Clinical Practice (ICH- GCP) R6E2 requirements

An essential consideration of any cannabis clinical trial is the stability of the cannabis medicines and the robustness both of their supply chain and the methods used to assess their stability [54]. It is imperative that any medication under study is available via a reliable and continuous supply for the duration of the study and for any ethically approved post-study period. This is particularly important when utilizing plant-based sources that can have inherent variability compared to chemically-synthesized medicines of mainstream pharmaceutical products.

As the legal production of GMP-certified cannabis medicines that are suitable for clinical trials is limited to certain countries, securing appropriate supply may involve transportation across international and state borders. Export and import logistics, licensing, permits, and quarantine requirements may be a consideration to ensure adequate supply in a timely manner for the trial.

7. Engagement with industry

A diverse stakeholder cohort underpins all clinical trials. In cannabis research, most stakeholders—clinicians, researchers, regulatory bodies, and the medicinal cannabis industry—support the need for robust clinical evidence that informs the use of cannabis derived therapeutics. In Australia as in other countries, cooperation amongst stakeholders is essential to ensure the challenges associated with a complex regulatory environment are appropriately addressed. Furthermore, stakeholders have the responsibility of managing industry expectations and delivering a level of patient recruitment that leads to successful clinical trials as well as fostering more efficient and effective collaborations.

A lack of global consistency on quality standards presents a different challenge. Establishing collaborations and implementing common agreements with local industry provides a framework to share knowledge especially when accessing the GMP cannabis medicines produced in Australia. Moreover, importation of products for clinical trials requires authorization, first from the country to which the product will be imported and subsequently from the country from which the product will be exported. Industry stakeholders may be highly responsive and supportive, but response timelines of regulators on both ends of the importing process can be prolonged and unreliable and may impact continuity of supply for longer-term trials. In addition, the requirement to comply with local standards that are geographically specific and often unique to cannabis medicines, means that the supplier must be both willing and capable of meeting those standards. In practical terms, this requirement can constrain a research team to source cannabis medicines only from companies with an established local operation with experience in the current regulations. Without this experience the impost of ensuring compliance shall fall either on the supplier or the research project and is likely to be cost-prohibitive.

8. Conclusion

The design of clinical trials for cannabis medicines is a complex process. Before embarking on a clinical trial, researchers need to have a clear understanding of the potential therapeutic benefit cannabis medicines may have. This understanding will inform the selection of cannabis product, the formulation of the product and the dose to be tested. Researchers must also be aware of regulations that are applicable where the research is to be undertaken as well as regulations that may be imposed at the source of the cannabis product. The phytochemical consistency of plant-derived products can be solidified with further research and may assist the approval of additional botanical products to the cannabis medicines market, increasing options for clinicians and patients, as plant-based products may be preferred to chemically-synthesized or bioengineered medicines [55]. Importantly, collaborations with industry are key to the successful outcome of cannabis medicines clinical trials. Without significant investment and sponsorship of clinical trials, the ability to generate quality data will be limited and the evidence for cannabis medicines to be registered as therapeutics lacking. Collaborations between researchers, industry and regulators, working together in sharing knowledge will generate high quality cannabis medicines research.

Acknowledgements

We would like to thank the members of the Australian Centre for Cannabinoid Clinical and Research Excellence (ACRE) Guidance Writing Group for Clinical Trials in Cannabinoids: Selection, Purchase and Supply of Cannabis Medicines as Study Drugs in Clinical Trials members Prof Janet Hardy (Mater Cancer Care Centre) and A/Prof Phillip Good (Mater Cancer Care Centre) for their contribution to the development of this paper.

Author Disclosure Statement

Dr Peter Galettis, Dr Rachel Galettis and Mrs Courtney Hill are part of the Australian Centre for Cannabinoid Clinical and Research Excellence (ACRE), which is funded through the National Health and Medical Research Council's Centres of Research Excellence Program. ACRE also receives funding through NSW Health's Clinical Cannabis Medicines Program.

John Barlow is a consultant to Applied Cannabis Research.

Jaroslav Boublik is Chief Science Officer of LeafCann Group Pty Ltd, a privately held Australian federally licensed medicinal cannabis production company.

Myfanwy Graham is funded through NSW Health's Clinical Cannabis Medicines Program.

Melinda Thompson is an alternate board member for the Medicinal Cannabis Industry Australia (MCIA)

Aaron Wong is Primary Investigator in a medicinal cannabis trial which is funded by the Victorian Cancer Agency.

SC, JSa, JS, PM, RR, LT, KW, & BZ – No competing financial interests exist

Author details

Peter Galettis[1,2]*, John Barlow[3], Jaroslav Boublik[4], Stefania Capra[5], Rachel Galettis[1,2], Myfanwy Graham[1,2,6], Courtney Hill[1,2], Paul Mavor[7], Jasminka Nikolajevic-Sarunac[8], Rosemary Richards[9], Janet Schloss[10], Melinda Thompson[11], Linda Truong[1,12,13], Berzenn Urbi[14,15], Katrina Weston-Green[1,16,17] and Aaron K. Wong[18,19,20]

1 Australian Centre for Cannabinoid Clinical and Research Excellence, The University of Newcastle, Newcastle, Australia

2 Centre for Drug Repurposing and Medicines Research, School of Medicine and Public Health, The University of Newcastle, Newcastle, Australia

3 Applied Cannabis Research, Sydney, Australia

4 LeafCann Group Pty Ltd, Adelaide, Australia

5 Department of Pharmacy, Royal Prince Alfred Hospital, Camperdown, Australia

6 NSW Cannabis Medicines Advisory Service, Newcastle, Australia

7 Health House International Pty Ltd, Perth, Australia

8 Investigational Drugs/Clinical Trials, Hunter New England Health, Pharmacy Department, John Hunter Hospital, Newcastle, Australia

9 Medicinal Cannabis Industry Australia, Sydney, Australia

10 National Centre for Naturopathic Medicine, Southern Cross University, Lismore, Australia

11 Source Certain International Limited, formerly AusCann Group Holdings Ltd, Perth, Australia

12 Department of Neurology, Sydney Children's Hospitals, Randwick, NSW, Australia

13 Faculty of Medicine, School of Women's and Children's Health, University of New South Wales, Sydney, Australia

14 Office for Research Governance and Development, Gold Coast Hospital and Health Service, Southport, Australia

15 School of Medicine, Griffith University, Southport, Australia

16 Faculty of Science Medicine and Health, Molecular Horizons and School of Medicines, University of Wollongong, School of Medicine, Wollongong, Australia

17 Illawarra Health and Medical Research Institute, Wollongong, Australia

18 Peter MacCallum Cancer Centre, Parkville, Australia

19 Royal Melbourne Hospital, Parkville, Australia

20 The University of Melbourne, Parkville, Australia

*Address all correspondence to: peter.galettis@newcastle.edu.au

References

[1] Morales P, Hurst DP, Reggio PH. Molecular targets of the phytocannabinoids: A complex picture. Progress in the Chemistry of Organic Natural Products. 2017;**103**:103-131

[2] Lucas CJ, Galettis P, Schneider J. The pharmacokinetics and the pharmacodynamics of cannabinoids. British Journal of Clinical Pharmacology. 2018;**84**(11):2477-2482

[3] Australian New Zealand Clinical Trials Registry. 2020. Available from: https://www.anzctr.org.au/

[4] U. S. National Library of Medicine [cited 25 September 2020]. Available from: https://clinicaltrials.gov/

[5] World Health Organisation. International Clinical Trials Registry Platform (ICTRP) [cited 25 September 2020]. Available from: https://www.who.int/ictrp/en/

[6] Mucke M, Weier M, Carter C, et al. Systematic review and meta-analysis of cannabinoids in palliative medicine. Journal of Cachexia, Sarcopenia and Muscle. 2018;**9**(2):220-234

[7] Lacey J, Schloss JM, Sinclair J, et al. A phase II double-blind, randomized clinical trial assessing the tolerability of two different ratios of cannabis in patients with glioblastoma multiforme (GBM). Journal of Clinical Oncology. 2020;**38**(suppl. 15):2530

[8] Hoch E, Niemann D, von Keller R, et al. How effective and safe is medical cannabis as a treatment of mental disorders? A systematic review. European Archives of Psychiatry and Clinical Neuroscience. 2019;**269**(1):87-105

[9] Laux LC, Bebin EM, Checketts D, et al. Long-term safety and efficacy of cannabidiol in children and adults with treatmentresistant Lennox-Gastaut syndrome or Dravet syndrome: Expanded access program results. Epilepsy Research. 2019;**154**:13-20

[10] Nielsen S, Germanos R, Weier M, et al. The use of Cannabis and cannabinoids in treating symptoms of multiple sclerosis: A systematic review of reviews. Current Neurology and Neuroscience Reports. 2018;**18**(2):8

[11] Lintzeris N, Bhardwaj A, Mills L, et al. Nabiximols for the treatment of cannabis dependence: A Randomized Clinical Trial. JAMA Internal Medicine. 2019;**179**(9):1242-1253

[12] Campbell G, Stockings E, Nielsen S. Understanding the evidence for medical cannabis and cannabis-based medicines for the treatment of chronic non-cancer pain. European Archives of Psychiatry and Clinical Neuroscience. 2019;**269**(1):135-144

[13] Badowski ME, Yanful PK. Dronabinol oral solution in the management of anorexia and weight loss in AIDS and cancer. Therapeutics and Clinical Risk Management. 2018;**14**:643-651

[14] Chow R, Valdez C, Chow N, et al. Oral cannabinoid for the prophylaxis of chemotherapy-induced nausea and vomiting-a systematic review and meta-analysis. Supportive Care in Cancer. 2020;**28**(5):2095-2103

[15] Hillen JB, Soulsby N, Alderman C, Caughey GE. Safety and effectiveness of cannabinoids for the treatment of neuropsychiatric symptoms in dementia: A systematic review. Therapeutic

Advances in Drug Safety. January 2019. DOI: 10.1177/2042098619846993

[16] Bruni N, Della Pepa C, Oliaro-Bosso S, et al. Cannabinoid delivery systems for pain and inflammation treatment. Molecules. 2018;**23**(10):2478

[17] Huestis MA. Pharmacokinetics and metabolism of the plant cannabinoids, delta9-tetrahydrocannabinol, cannabidiol and cannabinol. Handbook of Experimental Pharmacology. 2005;**168**:657-690

[18] Ahmed AI, van den Elsen GA, Colbers A, et al. Safety, pharmacodynamics, and pharmacokinetics of multiple oral doses of delta-9-tetrahydrocannabinol in older persons with dementia. Psychopharmacology. 2015;**232**(14):2587-2595

[19] Borgelt LM, Franson KL, Nussbaum AM, et al. The pharmacologic and clinical effects of medical Cannabis. Pharmacotherapy. 2013;**33**(2):195-209

[20] Stinchcomb AL, Valiveti S, Hammell DC, et al. Human skin permeation of Delta8-tetrahydrocannabinol, cannabidiol and cannabinol. The Journal of Pharmacy and Pharmacology. 2004;**56**(3):291-297

[21] Oh DA, Parikh N, Khurana V, et al. Effect of food on the pharmacokinetics of dronabinol oral solution versus dronabinol capsules in healthy volunteers. Clinical Pharmacology. 2017;**9**:9-17

[22] Karschner EL, Darwin WD, Goodwin RS, et al. Plasma cannabinoid pharmacokinetics following controlled oral delta9-tetrahydrocannabinol and oromucosal cannabis extract administration. Clinical Chemistry. 2011;**57**(1):66-75

[23] MacCallum CA, Russo EB. Practical considerations in medical cannabis administration and dosing. European Journal of Internal Medicine. 2018;**49**:12-19

[24] Khaiser M, Peng M, Ahrari S, et al. Medical cannabis dosing strategies in pain-related conditions: A scoping review of current literature. Journal of Pain Management. 2016;**9**:449-463

[25] Carter GT, Weydt P, Kyashna-Tocha M, et al. Medicinal cannabis: Rational guidelines for dosing. IDrugs. 2004;**7**(5):464-470

[26] Larsen C, Shahinas J. Dosage, efficacy and safety of cannabidiol administration in adults: A systematic review of human trials. Journal of Clinical Medical Research. 2020;**12**(3):129-141

[27] Devinsky O, Cross JH, Laux L, et al. Trial of cannabidiol for drug-resistant seizures in the Dravet Syndrome. The New England Journal of Medicine. 2017;**376**(21):2011-2020

[28] Novotna A, Mares J, Ratcliffe S, et al. A randomized, double-blind, placebo-controlled, parallel-group, enriched-design study of nabiximols* (Sativex(®), as add-on therapy, in subjects with refractory spasticity caused by multiple sclerosis. European Journal of Neurology. 2011;**18**(9):1122-1131

[29] Millar SA, Stone NL, Bellman ZD, et al. A systematic review of cannabidiol dosing in clinical populations. British Journal of Clinical Pharmacology. 2019;**85**(9):1888-1900

[30] Bergamaschi MM, Queiroz RH, Zuardi AW, et al. Safety and side effects of cannabidiol, a Cannabis sativa constituent. Current Drug Safety. 2011;**6**(4):237-249

[31] Kocis PT, Vrana KE. Delta-9-tetrahydrocannabinol and cannabidiol drug-drug interactions. Med Cannabis Cannabinoids. 2020;**3**(1):61-73

[32] Penn State University College of Medicine. Cannabinoid Drug-Drug Interactions [cited 28 September 2020]. Available from: https://sites.psu.edu/cannabinoid/

[33] Silva DA, Pate DW, Clark RD, et al. Influences of phytocannabinoids on drug-drug interactions and their clinical implications. Pharmacology & Therapeutics. 2020;**2020**:107621

[34] Gaston TE, Bebin EM, Cutter GR, et al. Interactions between cannabidiol and commonly used antiepileptic drugs. Epilepsia. 2017;**58**(9):1586-1592

[35] Hauser W, Finn DP, Kalso E, et al. European Pain Federation (EFIC) position paper on appropriate use of cannabis-based medicines and medical cannabis for chronic pain management. European Journal of Pain. 2018

[36] Weston-Green K, Clunas H, Jimenez NC. A review of the potential use of pinene and linalool as terpene-based medicines for brain health: Discovering Novel Therapeutics in the Flavours and Fragrances of Cannabis. Frontiers in Psychology. 2021;**12**(583211):1-15

[37] Therapeutic Goods Administration. Conforming with Therapeutic Goods (Standard for Medicinal Cannabis) (TGO 93) Order 2017 2019 [cited. Available from: https://www.tga.gov.au/conforming-therapeutic-goods-standard-medicinal-cannabis-tgo-93-order-2017

[38] U.S Food & Drug Administration. Cannabis and Cannabis-Derived Compounds: Quality Considerations for Clinical Research Guidance for Industry [Internet] [cited 21 September 2020]. Available from: https://www.fda.gov/media/140319/download

[39] U.S Food & Drug Administration. Clinical Trials Guidance Document [updated 21 January 2020; cited 22 September 2020]. Available from: https://www.fda.gov/regulatory-information/search-fda-guidance-documents/clinical-trials-guidance-documents

[40] European Medicines Agency. Clinical Trials in human medicines [cited 22 September 2020]. Available from: https://www.ema.europa.eu/en/human-regulatory/research-development/clinical-trials-human-medicines

[41] Therapeutic Goods Administration. Clinical Trials 2020 [updated 25 March 2020; cited. Available from: https://www.tga.gov.au/clinical-trials

[42] Therapeutic Goods Administration. Contacts for State/Territory medicines & poisons regulation units 2020 [cited 22 September 2020]. Available from: https://www.tga.gov.au/contacts-stateterritory-medicines-poisons-regulation-units

[43] Therapeutic Goods Administration. PE009, the PIC/S guide to GMP for medicinal products [Internet] [cited 24 August 2020]. Available from: https://www.tga.gov.au/sites/default/files/pe009-pics-guide-gmp-medicinal-products.pdf

[44] Therapeutic Goods Administration. Medicinal cannabis manufacture 2019 [cited. Available from: https://www.tga.gov.au/book-page/investigational-medicinal-products-annex-13-0

[45] Therapeutic Goods Administration. Australian clinical trial handbook [Internet] Version 2.2. [cited 22 September 2020]. Available from: https://www.tga.gov.au/sites/default/files/australian-clinical-trial-handbook.pdf

[46] Therapeutic Goods Administration. Microbiological quality of medicinal cannabis products 2020 [cited 22 September 2020]. Available from: https://www.tga.gov.au/publication/microbiological-quality-medicinal-cannabis-products

[47] Therapeutic Goods Administration. Guidance for TGO 101 2020 [cited 22 September 2020]. Available from: https://www.tga.gov.au/publication/guidance-tgo-101

[48] Therapeutic Goods Administration. Good manufacturing practice - an overview 2017 [cited 22 September 2020]. Available from: https://www.tga.gov.au/good-manufacturing-practice-overview

[49] Therapeutic Goods Administration. Medicinal cannabis manufacture [Internet] Version 1.0. [cited 22 September 2020]. Available from: https://www.tga.gov.au/sites/default/files/medicinal-cannabis-manufacture.pdf

[50] Therapeutic Goods Administration. Scheduling of medicines & poisons [Internet] [cited 07 August 2020]. Available from: https://www.tga.gov.au/scheduling-medicines-poisons

[51] NSW Health. Schedule 8 Cannabis Medicines and Unregistered Schedule 8 Medicines [Internet] IB2019_041. [cited 24 August 2020]. Available from: https://www1.health.nsw.gov.au/pds/ActivePDSDocuments/IB2019_041.pdf

[52] Alcohol and Drug Foundation. Medicinal cannabis / medicinal cannabinoids [cited. Available from: https://cdn.adf.org.au/media/documents/Medicinal-Cannabis-Fact-Sheet-FINAL.pdf

[53] Australian Government Department of Health Office of Drug Control. Manufacturers 2020 [cited 22 September 2020]. Available from: https://www.odc.gov.au/manufacturers-1

[54] Pacifici R, Marchei E, Salvatore F, et al. Evaluation of cannabinoids concentration and stability in standardized preparations of cannabis tea and cannabis oil by ultra-high performance liquid chromatography tandem mass spectrometry. Clinical Chemistry and Laboratory Medicine. 2017;**55**(10):1555-1563

[55] Kruger DJ, Kruger JS. Medical cannabis users' comparisons between medical cannabis and mainstream medicine. Journal of Psychoactive Drugs. 2019;**51**(1):31-36

Chapter 3

Perspective Chapter: Endocannabinoids in Renal Physiology – From Tissue Homeostasis to Precision Medicine

Gloria M.R.S. Grelle, Luzia S. Sampaio and Marcelo Einicker-Lamas

Abstract

Body homeostasis is fully dependent on the different physiological systems working together in an orchestrated way. Different hormones, autacoids, and other bioactive molecules are known to play a role in the modulation of such events, either during a normal response to different stimuli or upon any harmful condition that will impact tissue or organ. The kidneys are very important for whole body homeostasis as they are responsible for the control of blood pressure, maintenance of the water compartments volume and composition, detoxification, reabsorption, pH regulation, and even some hormone production. Here we will discuss the ability of cannabinoids (phyto- or endocannabinoids) as modulators of renal physiology, which may open new perspectives for the development of new therapeutic drugs or the discovery of new patterns of endocannabinoids that may be explored as biomarkers for nephropathies or kidney repair toward precision medicine initiatives.

Keywords: anandamide, 2-AG, CB1 receptor, kidney, omics

1. Introduction

Despite their relatively small volume compared with other organs, the kidneys receive up to 20–25% of cardiac output, being this significant blood supply, the basis of most of the organ functions. Kidneys are not only "filters" that remove useless metabolites and other undesirable substances from the plasma, directing them for excretion resulting in urine production. The kidneys participate in key events for the body's homeostasis such as regulating the volume and tonicity of the body's fluid compartments, maintaining acid-base balance, controlling blood pressure, reabsorption of key solutes (glucose, amino acids, and bicarbonate), and regulating the body's water balance and production of hormones such as erythropoietin and calcitriol. The anatomical functional organization of the kidneys establishes a perfect harmony between structure and function that makes these organs quite complex and precise in their physiology.

 IntechOpen

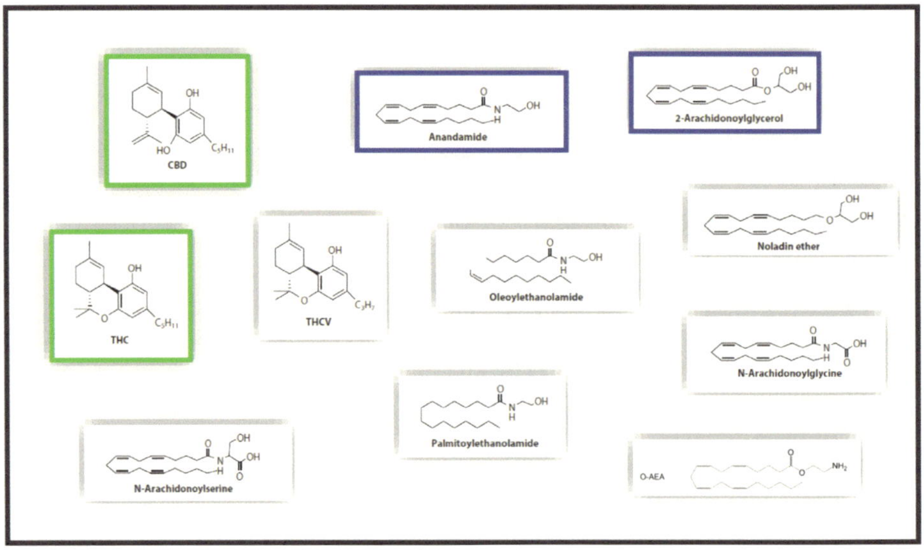

Figure 1.
Chemical structures of the principal cannabinoids: Highlighted in green, the phytocannabinoids: CBD, Cannabidiol; THC, Δ^9-tetrahydrocannabinol. Highlighted in blue, the most studied endocannabinoids: AEA, arachidonoyl ethanolamine (anandamide); 2-AG, 2-arachidonoyl glycerol. Not highlighted, some other identified endocannabinoids with physiological relevance in different tissues and organs.

In the last century, the research on the potential medical use of plant cannabinoids emerges with some important hallmarks for the field: (i) the identification and isolation of cannabidiol (CBD), Δ^9 tetrahydrocannabinol (THC), and many other cannabidiol derivatives; (ii) the identification, isolation, and pharmacological characterization of the cannabinoid receptors (mainly CB1, CB2, and TRPV1[1]); and also (iii) as receptors should be present in the cells to trigger distinct cell signaling pathways through the action of endogenous bioactive molecules, the studies in the area allowed the identification and isolation of the so-called "endocannabinoids," an emerging class of lipidic molecules with a broad spectrum of action considering the widespread distribution of the cannabinoid receptors within the different tissues and physiological systems (**Figure 1**). Arachinodonoyl ethanolamide (anandamide) and 2-arachinodoyl glycerol (2-AG) are by far, the most studied and explored endogenous cannabinoids [1]. Endocannabinoid system (ECS) is known to participate in a variety of physiological and pathophysiological processes, as referred to in the literature where we can find reviews considering the pathways and involved enzymes for endocannabinoid synthesis and metabolism [2, 3]. Here, we will try to gather aspects of the experimental evidence involving the ECS and how it can interact with kidney tissue and function. We will try to bring to the scene the emerging potential of endocannabinoids as valuable biomarkers for different diseases, focusing on their relevance in renal physiology. This will add new candidates to the different growing lists of molecules (some are still not identified), which are being considered as potential biomarkers, a striking point in the precision medicine initiative [4]. It is worth mentioning that we will emphasize those endogenous molecules, which are

[1] The transient receptor potential vanilloid type 1 (TRPV1) is not only activated by their initially identified ligands capsaicin and endovanniloids, but also by the endocannabinoids, which includes TRPVs in the hall of potential targets for the development of new drugs.

naturally synthesized and metabolized by our body resulting in the already known different endocannabinoids. Once produced, these bioactive molecules are able to trigger different cell signaling cascades through the activation of their specific receptors that together with the different endocannabinoids, and the enzymes for synthesis and degradation constitute the ECS, which is very well studied for its actions on the nervous system, being more recently explored in peripheral tissues. Nowadays, the importance of phyto- and endocannabinoid as regulators of physiological processes in practically all organs besides the central nervous system is a reality [5]. Among the peripheral organs, the renal ECS is growing in interest due to the importance in physiology and pathophysiology events that are known to impact the whole body. Endocannabinoids are known to share many of their actions with the components of different plant extracts that are currently being clinically administrated to different patients in order to minimize different pathologies, from a common headache to the enigmatic progression of different cancers. This new avenue opened by the medical use of cannabis allows us to reinforce that everything will be developed in this chapter regarding endocannabinoids can, to a large extent, be considered for aspects of the recreative or medical use of cannabis and their active principles (cannabidiol and THC). Thus, phytocannabinoids can be either complementary or disruptive to the function of the renal ECS with functional consequences that are not yet fully understood.

In the following items, we will seek to present the identity of these signaling molecules, and what is known about their action in renal physiology or renal cells in culture, a fundamental point of any scientific research that underpins advances and applications for the clinic and the well-being of human beings. We will also consider here the importance of the development of efficient analytical methods that would help to analyze the pattern of endocannabinoids either in health or disease models, a broadened attempt to identify potential biomarkers for different nephropathies adding support to initiatives in precision medicine.

2. The endocannabinoid system (ECS) and renal physiology

There is substantial literature showing that ECS is present and active in the kidneys, where it plays an important modulatory role in tissue physiology, and therefore, whole body homeostasis. **Figure 2** shows that the occurrence of the key enzymes involved in their metabolism (MAGL and FAAH) and the endocannabinoid receptors, CB1, CB2, GPCR55, and TRPV1, is expressed in the renal tissue, arterioles, and the glomeruli, which allow us to affirm that the ECS is present along the entire nephron structure [6]. The occurrence of these ECS elements shows that the renal tissue is not only capable of local synthesizing and remodeling the renal endocannabinoids pattern, but also processes different endocannabinoids and intermediates from other origins when they reach the kidneys through the blood supply. To illustrate this premise, the detection of anandamide and 2-arachidonoyl glycerol (2-AG) are well documented within the kidney tissue [7, 8].

In renal tissue, to date, there are few studies showing the actions of phyto- and/or endocannabinoids, and the most complete studies available were carried out in animal models. These studies were able to describe important events, such as the effect caused by anandamide on the renal vascular endothelium [9] and, the reduction of glomerular filtration rate by promoting vasorelaxation in afferent and efferent arterioles [10]. In addition, studies show that the administration of anandamide

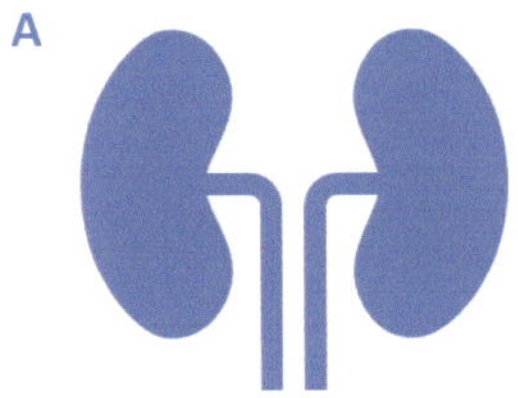

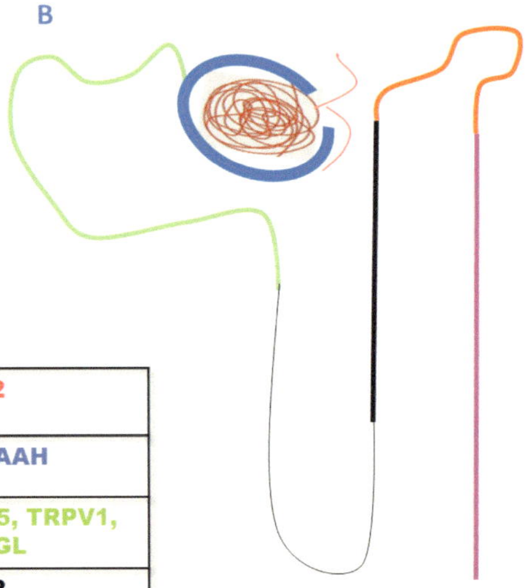

ARTERIOLES	CB1, CB2
GLOMERULUS	CB1, CB2, FAAH
PROXIMAL TUBULE	CB1, CB2, GPCR55, TRPV1, FAAH, MAGL
HENLE'S LOOP	CB1, CB2
DISTAL TUBULE	CB1, TRPV1, FAAH
COLLECTING DUCT	CB1, TRPV1, FAAH

Figure 2.
Endocannabinoid receptors and metabolizing enzymes within the nephron: renal system (A) is responsible for different key functions in body's homeostasis, such as the control of blood pressure, maintenance of the acid/basic balance and control the volume and composition of the liquid compartments. Each kidney possesses more than a million of functional units called nephrons (B), which are divided in specific segments: glomerulus, proximal tubule, Henle's Loop, distal tubule and collecting duct. The different components of the ECS were identified in the different nephron segments or arterioles as depicted in the table, according to the color code used. Abbreviations: CB1, CB2 and GPCR55, Cannabinoid receptors; TRPV1, transient receptor potential vanilloid type 1; FAAH, fatty acid amide hydrolase; MAGL, monoacylgliceryl lipase.

in the renal medulla of rats is able to promote a decrease in blood pressure through interaction with the CB1 cannabinoid receptor and an increase in urine volume due to interaction with TRPV1 receptors [11].

Activation of the CB2 receptor protected the kidney against the harmful effects caused by the administration of the anticancer drug cisplatin (also used in an animal model of nephrotoxicity), attenuating the characteristic inflammation [12]. CBD was also effective in minimizing the kidney injury induced by the ischemia/reperfusion model in mice/rats, by diminishing the harmful effects of either oxidative and nitrosative stress, and also reducing pro-inflammatory signals, as previously referred to the cisplatin injury [13, 14]. The importance of the renal ECS was also explored in diabetic renal disease, where it had been shown that endocannabinoid receptors can play an important role in either the worsening or the recovery of renal function, since CB1 activation is associated with the progression of the lesion, while CB1 inhibition together with CB2 activation would have an important protective role in this disease [15, 16].

Despite its potential benefits for different diseases, little is known about the use of phytocannabinoids and the impact of the plant-derived cannabinoids (mainly CBD and THC) on modulating renal function and treating renal pathologies. There are few clinical studies using cannabinoids and/or medical use of cannabis that take into account the repercussion on kidney function of human patients.

Anandamide (AEA), the first endocannabinoid described as showing a modulatory action in central and peripheral tissues, was the first element of the ECS that was characterized in the kidneys [9]. Actually, it is almost established that the renal production of anandamide appears to occur in different cell types, and most interestingly, it was observed that the medullary region produces higher levels of this endocannabinoid when compared with the renal cortex. It was also further described that other endocannabinoids, including 2-AG, are also synthesized in renal tissue [17, 18].

Physiology and pharmacodynamics study techniques, such as the binding assay, were explored to first show that anandamide was a ligand in renal endothelial microvascular cells with an efficiency comparable to that of specific agonists for CB1/CB2 cannabinoid receptors, as the synthetic cannabinoid CP55940, thus including anandamide in the hall of cannabinoid receptor agonists within the renal tissue. Indeed, the administration of exogenous anandamide has been shown to modulate the levels of released norepinephrine from renal sympathetic nerves [9]. From this milestone work, it became suggestive that the kidney tissue of mammals could present an active ECS that would be an important part of the maintenance and control of renal physiology, which highlighted a brand-new avenue for research focused on the effects of endocannabinoids in renal physiology and pathophysiology.

Regarding the expression, location, and functionality of cannabinoid receptors, the presence of CB1 receptor occurs in several renal regions, in the tubular segments of the nephrons, specifically in the proximal tubules, distal tubules, and intercalated cells of the collecting duct. In addition, CB1 receptor expression was also found in afferent and efferent arterioles and glomeruli, as well as in various renal cell subtypes, such as mesangial cells and podocytes (**Figure 2**). Likewise, the expression of CB2 receptors, although thought to be predominantly related to immune cells, has also been demonstrated in kidney tissue to be localized in podocytes, proximal tubule cells, and mesangial cells [7]. The CB2 receptor also appears to play an important role in the regulation of renal hemodynamics, as the work by Pressly and colleagues showed that the administration of a selective synthetic agonist for CB2 was able to increase renal cortical blood flow and also promote direct vasodilation of afferent arterioles when they were perfused alone [19].

The effects of anandamide and other cannabinoids on renal hemodynamics suggest that the renal ECS would be able to play a role in the regulation of blood pressure. This should involve a mechanism dependent on CB1 receptor activation, resulting in diuretic effects (increase in urinary flow without change in sodium excretion) probably acting on renal innervation [11]. It was also demonstrated that TRPV1 receptor is an important target for modulating renal hemodynamics, sodium, and water excretion, being precisely expressed in the sympathetic fibers of the renal innervation [20]. Indeed, activation of TRPV1 in the kidney by its exogenous agonist capsaicin produces diuresis and natriuresis mediated in part by a marked increase in glomerular filtration rate and activation of renal innervation. Activation of the TRPV1 receptor provides a protective mechanism against the elevation of blood pressure induced by high salt intake; however, the assessment of the specific contribution of anandamide-induced TRPV1 receptor modulation is complicated by the various other sensory stimuli capable of activating this receptor [8]. The diuretic effect of endogenous and exogenous cannabinoids was most extensively investigated in the work by Paronis and colleagues [21]. Using Sprague-Dawley rats as a model, the work showed that cannabinoids, including anandamide itself (meta-anandamide, a more stable synthetic analog, often used also), the phytocannabinoid THC, and the synthetic cannabinoids WIN55,212-2, AM2389, and AM4054, thus showing that cannabinoids of different classes are able to increase diuresis in a dose-dependent manner. Strikingly, the diuretic effects produced by THC, WIN55,212-2, AM2389, and AM4054 were comparable to that of the loop diuretic furosemide, known to be the chosen drug of the most potent class of diuretics.

There is substantial information in the literature ascribing anandamide an important role in the regulation of renal hemodynamics, either through its direct action or through the generation of active metabolites, such as prostamide E2, with equal diuretic and natriuretic effects [17]. The diuretic effect implies the possible modulation of different ion transporters that are present in the different nephron segments, being the Na^+/K^+-ATPase, the main pump involved in Na^+ reabsorption and in the maintenance of the Na^+ gradient that is crucial for other solutes reabsorption or secretion. Thus, a direct correlation between augmented diuresis and Na^+ excretion is a clue that would include the endocannabinoids in the hall of the bioactive molecules with potential action on the different ion transporters.

This issue was explored in vitro, using porcine proximal tubule cells (LLC-PK1) that are related to the most cortical region of the kidney. The authors showed that the activation of the CB1 receptor through the addition of a synthetic cannabinoid agonist, WIN55,212-2, was able to increase sodium reabsorption as a result of increased Na^+/K^+-ATPase activity present in the basolateral membrane of these cells [22]. Conversely, it was also demonstrated that anandamide reduced the sodium reabsorption by the proximal tubule Na^+/H^+ exchanger and the $Na^+/K^+/2Cl^-$ cotransporter present in the thick ascending limb of the Henle's loop [23]. Unfortunately, few studies have been carried out in humans to date, so little is known about the applicability of cannabinoids and their impact on renal physiology, especially with regard to the impact on renal function over the years. Meanwhile, one of the studies in humans is an extensive one that followed 5115 volunteers over a long period (25 years) in order to assess whether recreational cannabis use had implications for adult kidney function. Overall, although a modest association was identified between greater cannabis exposure and lower glomerular filtration rate (cystatin C assay) among volunteers, the results were inconclusive and did not demonstrate any significant association between cannabis use and changes in glomerular filtration rate or prevalent albuminuria [24]. Besides, recreational use of synthetic cannabinoids appears to have a negative impact on kidney function. Some case reports in recent years have pointed to a direct correlation between the use of synthetic cannabinoids (used recreationally, often through the use of e-cigarettes) and severe acute kidney disease, but without any mechanistic understanding of this correlation [25]. In summary, the case reports only state that patients who used these synthetic substances developed significant hypertension, agitation, respiratory failure (some required intubation), pulmonary hypertension, and acute kidney injury, with high levels of creatinine and urea. The pathological mechanism of acute kidney disease remains unclear, but it was suggested that would be acute tubular necrosis and/or acute interstitial nephritis, as evidenced by biopsies performed in patients from some of the case report studies. Although the above-mentioned harmful effects attributed to the recreational use of synthetic cannabinoids, the emerging potential use of endocannabinoids as well as phytocannabinoids as modulators of the renal machinery, would allow the development of new therapeutical strategies, products, and clinical procedures for the treatment of renal and non-renal pathologies [26, 27].

2.1 Cannabinoids as a therapeutical perspective for different nephropathies

The functional relevance of ECS in renal tissue is credited by previously mentioned findings, with a direct impact mainly on the regulation of renal hemodynamics, as well as on the dysregulation of this function in pathological states, such as in renal disease associated with acute kidney disease and diabetic renal disease [28]. The endpoint of these pathological conditions is chronic kidney disease, which presents marked proteinuria, inflammation, fibrosis, and renal failure, converging to dialysis and even transplantation. There are no efficient treatments for the different nephropathies, so any initiative to develop new clinical protocols, here included those exploring the versatility of the endocannabinoids and phytocannabinoids, should be strongly encouraged.

2.1.1 Acute kidney injury

Acute kidney injury (AKI) describes a sudden loss of kidney function that is determined on the basis of increased serum creatinine levels (a marker of kidney excretory function) and reduced urinary output (oliguria; a quantitative marker of urine production) and is limited to a duration of 7 days. We will not discuss the pathophysiology of AKI as there are substantial literature detailing it [29]. AKI can occur due to a number of factors, such as the onset of a sepsis process, exposure to nephrotoxins, and organ hypoperfusion due to ischemia. In fact, ischemia-reperfusion (IR) injury is one of the most common forms of AKI and involves a complex series of cellular changes that can lead to damage and death of tubular cells and loss of renal function in the most severe cases. Regulation of renal blood flow dynamics is necessary to preserve glomerular filtration rate during IR-induced AKI critical in damage propagation and kidney recovery [19]. To understand the mechanisms by which the endocannabinoid system is correlated with the events that lead to AKI, many animal models are used; among these, cisplatin-induced nephrotoxicity and the IR lesion induction technique.

Using the IR injury model in mice, Feizi and co-workers showed that pretreatment with both selective CB1 and CB2 receptor agonists was able to protect kidney tissue from IR damage, suggesting an important role for ECS to protect the kidneys from possible cellular damage caused by IR [30]. In this work, it is important to emphasize that the treatment performed with synthetic cannabinoids was prior to the induction of the IR lesion, which implies a protective and not a curative effect. In another study, Sampaio and colleagues used the IR lesion in both in vitro and in vivo models in Wistar rats, demonstrating that the lesion leads a significant reduction in the anandamide levels, as well as in the expression of CB1 receptors in the renal cortex region [18]. Another study using the IR injury in mice showed that renal cell damage and characteristic biochemical changes were associated with increased levels of 2-AG in all renal tissue [31]. The relation between kidney disease and ECS was also explored by Sampaio and co-workers, who had demonstrated in rats that after IR injury there was a significative inhibition in the Na^+/K^+-ATPase activity present in the basolateral membrane of proximal tubule cells, which was fully reverted in the experimental group that was treated with the synthetic cannabinoid WIN55,212,-2 immediately after the IR injury [18]. The cannabinoid agonist led to the recovery of sodium transport, through a pathway dependent on the activation of the CB1 receptor. This is in agreement with previous work from the group and allowed them to suggest that the ECS plays an important role in the re-establishment of Na^+ reabsorption and consequence, other solutes, such as glucose and amino acids in the renal proximal tubule, since the normal Na^+/K^+-ATPase activity in these tubular cells directly impacts all solute transport in this tubular segment as it restores or keeps the Na^+ gradient, which is the driven-force for different secondary active transporters above mentioned [32].

In 2012, a pioneer study was carried out to evaluate the potential protective effect of CBD, in an IR model injury in rats. The intravenous administration of CBD (before and after the IR procedure) was able to protect kidney tissue from injury-associated damage [14]. Authors showed that IR promoted changes in different histological and clinical biochemical markers, such as azotemia and uremia (increased levels of toxic nitrogenous compounds in the bloodstream) associated with a significant decrease in renal glutathione levels. CBD treatment significantly attenuated the observed harmful alterations in the biochemical parameters evaluated. Furthermore, the histopathological analysis showed that CBD improved the healthy condition of the renal tissue, significantly reducing the expression of inducible nitric oxide synthase (related to macrophage infiltration and inflammation), tumor necrosis factor-alpha, cyclooxygenase-2, and caspase-3 [14]. These findings were further confirmed by the work of Baban and colleagues using a similar model of injury. These authors showed that the treatment with CBD protected the renal tissue from damage, restoring renal blood flow, and serum creatinine levels. It was also observed that the phytocannabinoid was able to reduce neutrophil infiltration and inflammatory signals [33].

One of the main pharmacological targets of CBD is the anandamide-degrading enzyme, fatty acid amino hydrolase (FAAH). This important observation allows us to postulate that along their own beneficial effects, CBD would inhibit anandamide degradation, leading to increased levels of this endocannabinoid, which plays an important role in renal tissue homeostasis. Another hypothesis would be the action of CBD on TRPV1 receptors, which, plays a role in the maintenance of renal hemodynamics.

Although rare, other studies also sought to investigate the possible role of cannabinoid receptors in the IR model of AKI. Zhou and colleagues showed that blockage of the CB2 receptor decreases the fibrosis cascade, one of the hallmarks after IR injury both in vitro and in vivo. Agonist administration and/or CB2 overexpression was directly associated with increased synthesis of extracellular matrix proteins, such as smooth muscle alpha-actin and fibronectin, early markers of fibrosis. It was also shown that treatment with transforming growth factor beta 1 (TGFβ-1), an important pro-fibrotic cytokine, was related to increased CB2 expression. In this work, the group tested a new synthetic drug, which acts as a CB2 antagonist, and they were able to demonstrate how the administration of this cannabinoid reduced inflammation and fibrosis in animals subjected to IR injury [34].

In 2009, a study using cisplatin injury model of AKI, showed that CBD attenuated tissue damage and the expression of enzymes involved in oxidative processes, inflammation, necrosis, and renal apoptosis, in mice, associating this phytocannabinoid with a marked improvement in renal function [13]. The treatment with CBD was performed in mice 1 hour before the administration of cisplatin, a procedure repeated for 10 days. CBD largely attenuated the symptoms induced by cisplatin, mainly in terms of the increased expression of enzymes that generate reactive oxygen species (NOX4 and NOX1). It also decreased the cisplatin-induced inflammatory response, decreasing the levels of pro-inflammatory cytokines such as TNF-alpha and IL-1β, being such effects probably associated with the already reported antioxidant function of CBD. Further, Mukhopadhyay and colleagues using the same animal model for AKI showed that CB1 receptor activation plays a central role in the progression of kidney injury. The lesion caused by cisplatin was associated with an increase in renal anandamide levels, activation of signaling pathways involved with cell death, oxidative stress, leukocyte infiltration into the renal tissue, and inflammation, in addition to impaired renal function, with an increase in serum creatinine and urea levels [35].

Both the genetic deletion and the pharmacological inhibition of CB1 receptors with the use of the antagonists AM281 or SR141716 markedly attenuated cisplatin-induced renal dysfunction, but were not able to prevent the lesion and its characteristics, thus demonstrating that CB1 may play an important role in the progression of nephrotoxicity-induced AKI. The CB2 receptor, on the other hand, seems to behave in the opposite way, since it was shown, in the same model of cisplatin-induced renal injury that the use of a synthetic and selective CB2 agonist was able to attenuate the inflammatory response, oxidative stress, cell damage and improved renal function in animals [35], evidencing an important effect of the CB2 receptor in attenuating damage in this injury model.

2.1.2 Diabetic kidney disease

Most complications of diabetes are associated with pathological changes in the vascular endothelium wall. The most common macrovascular complication of diabetes is atherosclerosis, which increases the risk of myocardial infarction, stroke, and peripheral arterial disease; while microvascular complications underlie nephropathy, retinopathy, and peripheral neuropathy. Thus, diabetic kidney disease (DKD), initially referred to as diabetic nephropathy, is one of the main causes of kidney failure. In the diabetic patient, hyperglycemia stimulates the generation of reactive oxygen species, which ultimately leads (by several pathways) to DKD, characterized by mesangial and tubular cell hypertrophy, glomerular basement membrane thickening, and glomerular sclerosis [36]. DKD markers are increased glomerular permeability to proteins and excessive accumulation of extracellular matrix in the mesangium, eventually resulting in glomerulosclerosis and damage to the tubular epithelium due to increased filtered glucose load that results in osmotic effect, tubular cell death, increased urinary flux and progressive renal failure [15].

In studies using models of type I diabetes, such as the administration of streptozotocin or using spontaneously diabetic mice, it was demonstrated that the renal tissue of these animals showed a significant increase in the expression of the CB1 receptor, mainly in podocytes. In animals that received treatment with a synthetic CB1 antagonist, a significant reduction in albuminuria was observed, as well as a recovery in the expression of glomerular proteins associated with the proper functioning of the renal filtration barrier, such as nephrin, an important fact since in both human and experimental DKD there is a reduction in nephrin expression. Studies in patients with microalbuminuria have shown that downregulation of this protein occurs at an early stage of the disease [15, 37]. The involvement of the CB2 receptor in this model was also investigated, which shows a decrease in the expression in the glomerulus, and since diabetic mice induced by streptozotocin and treated for 14 weeks with AM1241, a synthetic selective agonist for CB2, an improvement in renal function with concomitant restoration of nephrin expression levels and reduction in the glomerular monocytes infiltration, observations that were also present in the study using animals with selective genetic deletion of CB2, showing that the absence of this receptor induces an even more severe renal damage condition in response to diabetes [16, 38]. In the aforementioned animal model, the levels of endocannabinoids were determined in the renal cortex and those of 2-AG were reduced in diabetic animals. In the same work, CB2 expression was also studied in human patients and cultured podocytes, showing that the CB2 receptor was less expressed in renal biopsies from diabetic patients, suggesting that CB2 activation is involved in both albuminuria and the loss of podocyte proteins that act on the stability of the glomerular filtration barrier. Therefore, this receptor would play a protective effect in patients with DKD [16]. Interestingly, when a combined treatment using the CB2 agonist AM1241 and the CB1 receptor antagonist AM6545, in streptozotocin-induced animal model of diabetes, resulted in a better prognostic than that observed using the usual monotherapies, abolishing albuminuria, monocyte infiltration and inflammation, tubular injury, and markedly reducing renal fibrosis [39].

The ECS modulatory action in models of type I diabetes was also confirmed in different animal models of renal disease associated with type II diabetes, in which animals showed an increase in the expression of CB1 in the renal glomerulus, an increase in albuminuria, a reduction in the glomerular filtration rate and nephrin expression, monocyte infiltration and inflammation, in addition to the activation of the renin-angiotensin system. Treatment with both CB1 antagonists and CB2 receptor agonists promotes significant improvement in these studied renal parameters [40, 41].

2.1.3 Chronic kidney disease

Chronic kidney disease (CKD) is an irreversible condition that affects millions of people around the world. Regardless of its initial cause, CKD is the final stage of replacement of functional kidney tissue by altered extracellular matrix proteins, characterizing renal fibrosis that almost completely limits the functionality of kidney tissue. To date, there are no therapeutic options available to prevent progression and treat both renal fibrosis and chronic kidney disease [42].

In this context, a key role of the CB1 receptor in the development of renal fibrosis was already described, using both human patient samples and the animal model of unilateral ureteral obstruction [42]. In mice, through molecular biology assays and bioinformatics resources, the CNR1 gene, which encodes the CB1 receptor, was one of the genes with the most altered expression in fibrotic kidneys. Immunohistochemical assays revealed that CB1 receptor expression increased dramatically in the renal fibrosis model and that the receptor was highly expressed in renal tubules, parenchyma, and glomerulus. These results were accompanied by a significant increase in CB2 receptor expression, 2-AG levels, and a reduction in anandamide levels. In pharmacological trials, treatment with the specific synthetic CB2 antagonist was shown to retard the development of fibrosis, while the CB2 agonist JWH133 attenuated renal fibrogenesis. These reported results add more evidence to the view that cannabinoid receptors may have antagonistic effects on renal tissue.

CKD also becomes an evident problem in kidney transplanted patients. The progressive and inevitable impairment of renal graft function remains the primary cause of graft loss, where such impairment is due to the replacement of functional renal tissue by extracellular matrix proteins, mainly collagens, leading to both interstitial fibrosis and tubular atrophy, accompanied by glomerulosclerosis. In a study that analyzed 26 patients, CB1 receptor expression levels were investigated on the day of transplantation, 3 months and 12 months after surgery [43]. The data revealed an increase in the expression of CB1 from the 3rd month on in grafts that presented functional impairment, thus being correlated with the onset and progression of renal fibrosis. The CB1 receptor was expressed mainly in proximal and distal tubular epithelial cells, arteries, and vascular smooth muscle cells of arterioles, in infiltrated inflammatory cells and glomeruli, mainly in podocytes.

3. Endocannabinoids as emerging biomarkers for kidney diseases: a precision medicine initiative

The mechanisms that promote and lead to kidney disease are being quickly elucidated due to research progress in Nephrology. Both genetic variation and metabolic changes caused by interactions with xenobiotics and lifestyle are being understood at the level of how they can affect predisposition and disease progression.

Precision medicine is one of the objectives of this research progress in different areas including nephrology, in which the patient's management is adapted according to the mechanisms underlying their disease aiming for maximal therapeutic success. The purpose of precision medicine is to characterize diseases based on the mechanisms involved in their pathophysiology and, thus, segregate patients and direct them to the best treatment. This is because there might be multiple pathways for the same phenotype and therapeutic strategies specific based on a single cell pathway or process may not be successful if applied to individuals differentially impacted in that specific illness. Therefore, the goal of precision medicine is to determine the right drug, in the right dose, for the right patient, at the right time.

Biomarkers are the basis of precision medicine, as they allow classifying individuals into subpopulations that differ in their susceptibility to a disease or in their response to a particular treatment. The term "biomarker," short for "biological marker," refers to a broad category of biological characteristics used to examine normal biological or pathological processes and responses to therapeutic or prophylactic interventions that can be accurately and reproducibly measured.

A good biomarker must link disease pathogenic mechanisms (endotypes) to visible properties (phenotypes), be reproducible, easy to measure and cost-effective, and be related to a clinical outcome. The role of biomarkers in the development of precision medicine offers an opportunity for technological developments aimed at improving human health and reducing healthcare costs. In this context, the Omics Sciences are highlighted, especially Metabolomics.

Metabolomics is the comprehensive study of the metabolome, that is, the set of biochemical compounds (or small molecules) present in cells, tissues, and body fluids. The study of metabolism at the global or "-omics" level is a rapidly growing field that has the potential to have a major impact on medical practice. The basis of metabolomics is the concept that a person's metabolic state provides a close representation of that individual's overall health status. This metabolic state reflects what has been encoded by the genome and modified by diet, environmental factors, and the gut microbiome, for example. The metabolic profile provides a differentiated reading of the biochemical status of normal physiology for various pathophysiology in a way that is often not seen from gene expression analysis.

Thus, the study of the metabolome is expected to reveal biochemical changes that reflect patterns of variation in well-being states and more accurately describe specific diseases and their progression, thus helping in the differential diagnosis (**Figure 3**). Through metabolomics, predictive, prognostic, diagnostic, and surrogate biomarkers of various disease states can be obtained, as well as information on the underlying molecular mechanisms of diseases, which will allow their sub-classification, and the stratification of patients based on the metabolic pathways affected. It also has the potential to reveal drug response biomarkers, providing an effective means to predict the variation in a subject's response to treatment and a means to monitor the response and recurrence of disease [44].

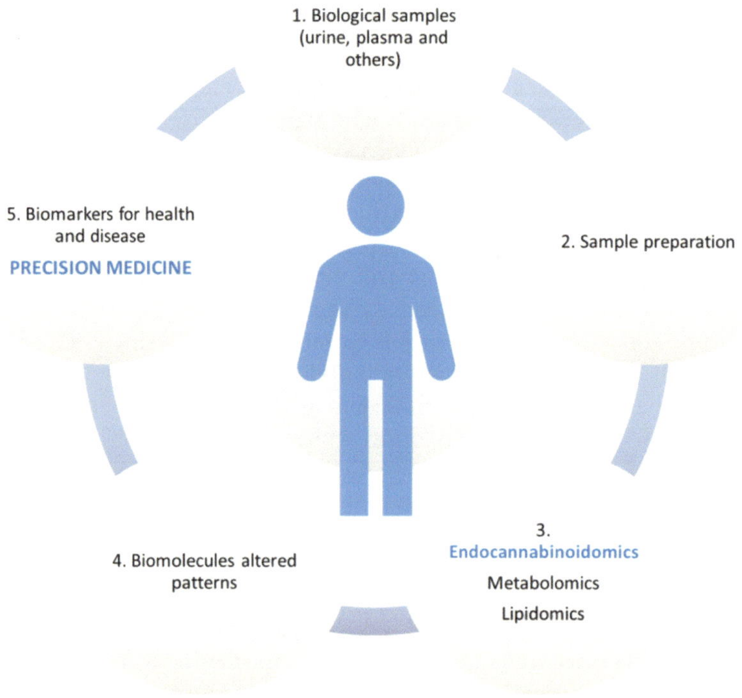

Figure 3.
Critical steps to stablish endocannabinoids as potential biomarkers for health and/or disease: This simply workflow allow us to identify different sequential steps that should be carried out in high quality conditions, from the pre-analytical phase to the conclusions obtained. We can assume the individual at the center, representing a healthy or a sick individual, which will be the donor (1) of any kind of biological sample, mainly urine and plasma. (2) the collected samples go further for extraction and preparation of the extracts to the different possible analysis. Here we assume that the samples will be submitted to different OMICs approaches such as Metabolomics, Lipidomics and the already mentioned in the literature, Endocannabinoidomics (3). The analysis will provide different biomolecules signatures that would be correlated to health or disease, according to the donor. This part of the analysis will allow us to identify altered patterns and specifically, altered molecular species for metabolites, lipids and also endocannabinoids (4). The results will be included in different biomolecules libraries that will help to group the different individuals, in their respective endotypes, based on the biomarkers found, which is a key point for the Precision Medicine Initiative (5).

Since Metabolomics is the study of small molecules, it encompasses the study of lipids (lipidomics) and, currently, mass spectrometry (MS) is the analytical technique that has been most used in these omics sciences. This is because MS allows accurate detection and quantification of molecules within a wide mass range. With the rapid development of MS in the detection of biomolecules, MS is emerging as an indispensable technology to accelerate research in the field of Precision Medicine [45].

In this context, the components of the ECS emerge as potential biomarkers for kidney diseases, whether for diagnostic, prognostic, or predictive applications, and also in an approach related to the discovery of new pharmacological targets. This is because the endocannabinoid system plays an important role in renal physiology, being a lipid cell signaling system that participates in different pathways. Alterations in this pathway can lead to the pathogenesis of both CKD and AKI. Recently, different anandamide-related molecules were identified in the brain, which may play a role in the normal or abnormal central nervous system physiology, according to their levels and distributions, leading to the molecular basis of human individual behavior, cognition, and temperamental differences [1]. This kind of endocannabinoid diversity may exist also in the peripheral organs, playing unknown roles in physiology and pathophysiology events. Therefore, the study of the endocannabinoid system at the level of the omics sciences is a promising area that may result in new therapies for different kidney diseases, thus contributing to the advancement of precision medicine in the field of nephrology.

4. Final remarks

In spite of the different experimental evidence shown here and elsewhere, it is inevitable to reinforce that to date, clinical studies with human patients have not yet been carried out in order to evaluate the use of cannabinoids for the treatment of chronic kidney disease, or for other kidney diseases, and even studies with the use of phytocannabinoids for these therapeutic purposes, even though preliminary tests and research in animals suggest a promising therapeutic use of phyto- and endocannabinoids for different nephropathies. It is also important to describe that the use of CBD, or even cannabis, for the treatment of other non-renal pathologies, does not seem to lead to any type of impairment of renal physiology and functioning, so, the medical use of phytocannabinoids does not lead to adverse effects on renal physiology. Obviously, specific monitoring of these aspects related to renal function and physiological events controlled by the kidneys should be better evaluated in long-term studies, since the bioavailability of exogenous cannabinoids in renal tissue can be quite significant, since kidneys are hyper perfused organs with a pleiade concentration of different receptors and other enzymes that integrate the Intra-Renal Endocannabinoid System itself.

Acknowledgements

Authors would like to acknowledge CNPq and Fundação Carlos Chagas de Amparo a Pesquisa do Estado do Rio de Janeiro for the financial support.

Conflict of interest

Authors would like to declare no conflict of interests.

Author details

Gloria M.R.S. Grelle, Luzia S. Sampaio and Marcelo Einicker-Lamas*
Laboratório de Biomembranas, Instituto de Biofísica Carlos Chagas Filho, Universidade Federal do Rio de Janeiro, Rio de Janeiro, Brazil

*Address all correspondence to: einicker@biof.ufrj.br

References

[1] Pacher P, Kogan NM, Mechoulam R. Beyond THC and endocannabinoids. Annual Review of Pharmacology and Toxicology. 2020;**60**:637-659. DOI: 10.1146/annurev-pharmtox-010818-021441

[2] Mechoulam R, Hanuš LO, Pertwee R, Howlett AC. Early phytocannabinoid chemistry to endocannabinoids and beyond. Nature Reviews. Neuroscience. 2014;**15**:757-764. DOI: 10.1038/nrn3811

[3] Maccarrone M. Missing pieces to the endocannabinoid puzzle. Trends in Molecular Medicine. 2020;**26**:263-272. DOI: 10.1016/j.molmed.2019.11.002

[4] Kratz D, Thomas D, Gurke R. Endocannabinoids as potential biomarkers: It's all about pre-analytics. Journal of Mass Spectrometry and Advances in the Clinical Lab. 2021;**22**:56-63. DOI: 10.1016/j.jmsacl.2021.11.001

[5] Szanda G, Mariscal IG, Jourdan T. Editorial: Multifaceted cannabinoids: Regulators of normal and pathological function in metabolic and endocrine organs. Frontiers in Endocrinology. 2022;**13**:1-2. DOI: 10.3389/fendo.2022.848050

[6] Barutta F, Bruno G, Mastrocola R, et al. The role of cannabinoid signaling in acute and chronic kidney diseases. Kidney International. 2018;**94**:252-258. DOI: 10.1016/j.kint.2018.01.024

[7] Chua JT, Argueta DA, Dipatrizio NV, et al. Endocannabinoid system and the kidneys: From renal physiology to injury and disease. Cannabis and Cannabinoid Research. 2019;**4**:10-20. DOI: 10.1089/can.2018.0060

[8] Ritter J, Li G, Xia M, Boini K. Anandamide and its metabolites: What are their roles in the kidney? Frontiers in Bioscience (Scholar Edition). 2016;**8**:264-277. DOI: 10.2741/s461

[9] Deutsch DG, Goligorsky MS, Schmid PC, et al. Production and physiological actions of anandamide in the vasculature of the rat kidney. The Journal of Clinical Investigation. 1997;**100**:1538-1546. DOI: 10.1172/JCI119677

[10] Koura Y, Ichihara A, Tada Y, et al. Anandamide decreases glomerular filtration rate through predominant vasodilation of efferent arterioles in rat kidneys. Journal of the American Society of Nephrology. 2004;**15**:1488-1494. DOI: 10.1097/01.ASN.0000130561.82631.BC

[11] Li J, Wang DH. Differential mechanisms mediating depressor and diuretic effects of anandamide. Journal of Hypertension. 2006;**24**:2271-2276. DOI: 10.1097/01.hjh.0000249706.42230.a8

[12] Mukhopadhyay P, Baggelaar M, Erdelyi K, et al. The novel, orally available and peripherally restricted selective cannabinoid CB2 receptor agonist LEI-101 prevents cisplatin-induced nephrotoxicity. British Journal of Pharmacology. 2016;**173**:446-458. DOI: 10.1111/bph.13338

[13] Pan H, Mukhopadhyay P, Rajesh M, et al. Cannabidiol attenuates cisplatin-induced nephrotoxicity by decreasing oxidative/nitrosative stress, inflammation, and cell death. The Journal of Pharmacology and Experimental Therapeutics. 2009;**328**:708-714. DOI: 10.1124/jpet.108.147181

[14] Fouad AA, Al-Mulhim AS, Jresat I. Cannabidiol treatment

ameliorates ischemia/reperfusion renal injury in rats. Life Sciences. 2012;**91**: 284-292. DOI: 10.1016/j.lfs.2012.07.030

[15] Barutta F, Corbelli A, Mastrocola R, et al. Cannabinoid receptor 1 blockade ameliorates albuminuria in experimental diabetic nephropathy. Diabetes. 2010;**59**:1046-1054. DOI: 10.2337/db09-1336

[16] Barutta F, Piscitelli F, Pinach S, et al. Protective role of cannabinoid receptor type 2 in a mouse model of diabetic nephropathy. Diabetes. 2011;**60**:2386-2396. DOI: 10.2337/db10-1809

[17] Ritter JK, Cao L, Xia M, et al. Production and actions of the anandamide metabolite prostamide E2 in the renal medulla. The Journal of Pharmacology and Experimental Therapeutics. 2012;**342**:770-779. DOI: 10.1124/jpet.112.196451

[18] Sampaio LS, Iannotti FA, Veneziani L, et al. Experimental ischemia/reperfusion model impairs endocannabinoid signaling and Na+/K+ ATPase expression and activity in kidney proximal tubule cells. Biochemical Pharmacology. 2018;**154**:482-491. DOI: 10.1016/j.bcp.2018.06.005

[19] Pressly JD, Soni H, Jiang S, et al. Activation of the cannabinoid receptor 2 increases renal perfusion. Physiological Genomics. 2019;**51**:90-96. DOI: 10.1152/physiolgenomics.00001.2019

[20] Wang HY, Wang Y, Zhang Y, et al. Crosslink between lipids and acute uveitis: A lipidomic analysis. International Journal of Ophthalmology. 2018;**11**:736-746 10.18240/ijo.2018.05.05

[21] Paronis CA, Thakur GA, Bajaj S, et al. Diuretic effects of cannabinoids. The Journal of Pharmacology and Experimental Therapeutics. 2013;**344**:8-14. DOI: 10.1124/jpet.112.199331

[22] Sampaio LS, Taveira Da Silva R, Lima D, et al. The endocannabinoid system in renal cells: Regulation of Na + transport by CB1 receptors through distinct cell signalling pathways. British Journal of Pharmacology. 2015;**172**:4615-4625. DOI: 10.1111/bph.13050

[23] Silva GB, Atchison DK, Juncos LI, García NH. Anandamide inhibits transport-related oxygen consumption in the loop of Henle by activating CB1 receptors. American Journal of Physiology-Renal Physiology. 2013;**304**:F376-F381. DOI: 10.1152/ajprenal.00239.2012

[24] Ishida JH, Auer R, Vittinghoff E, et al. Marijuana use and estimated glomerular filtration rate in young adults. Clinical Journal of the American Society of Nephrology. 2017;**12**:1578-1587. DOI: 10.2215/CJN.01530217

[25] Kazory A, Aiyer R. Synthetic marijuana and acute kidney injury: An unforeseen association. Clinical Kidney Journal. 2013;**6**:330-333. DOI: 10.1093/ckj/sft047

[26] Di Marzo V. New approaches and challenges to targeting the endocannabinoid system. Nature Reviews. Drug Discovery. 2018;**17**:623-639. DOI: 10.1038/nrd.2018.115

[27] Gregus AM, Buczynski MW. Druggable targets in endocannabinoid signaling. Advances in Experimental Medicine and Biology. 2020;**1274**:177-201. DOI: 10.1007/978-3-030-50621-6_8

[28] Tam J. The emerging role of the endocannabinoid system in the pathogenesis and treatment of kidney diseases. Journal of Basic and Clinical Physiology and Pharmacology.

2016;**27**:267-276. DOI: 10.1515/jbcpp-2015-0055

[29] Kellum JA, Romagnani P, Ashuntantang G, et al. Acute kidney injury. Nature Reviews Disease Primers. 2021;**7**:1-17. DOI: 10.1038/s41572-021-00284-z

[30] Feizi A, Jafari MR, Hamedivafa F, et al. The preventive effect of cannabinoids on reperfusion-induced ischemia of mouse kidney. Experimental and Toxicologic Pathology. 2008;**60**:405-410. DOI: 10.1016/j.etp.2008.04.006

[31] Moradi H, Oveisi F, Khanifar E, et al. Increased renal 2-arachidonoylglycerol level is associated with improved renal function in a mouse model of acute kidney injury. Cannabis and Cannabinoid Research. 2016;**1**:218-228. DOI: 10.1089/can.2016.0013

[32] Féraille E, Doucet A. Sodium-potassium-adenosinetriphosphatase-dependent sodium transport in the kidney: Hormonal control. Physiological Reviews. 2001;**81**:345-418. DOI: 10.1152/physrev.2001.81.1.345

[33] Baban B, Hoda N, Malik A, et al. Impact of cannabidiol treatment on regulatory T-17 cells and neutrophil polarization in acute kidney injury. American Journal of Physiology-Renal Physiology. 2018;**315**:F1149-F1158. DOI: 10.1152/ajprenal.00112.2018

[34] Zhou L, Zhou S, Yang P, et al. Targeted inhibition of the type 2 cannabinoid receptor is a novel approach to reduce renal fibrosis. Kidney International. 2018;**94**:756-772. DOI: 10.1016/j.kint.2018.05.023

[35] Mukhopadhyay P, Pan H, Rajesh M, et al. CB 1 cannabinoid receptors promote oxidative/nitrosative stress, inflammation and cell death in a murine nephropathy model. British Journal of Pharmacology. 2010;**160**:657-668. DOI: 10.1111/j.1476-5381.2010.00769.x

[36] Horvth B, Mukhopadhyay P, Hask G, Pacher P. The endocannabinoid system and plant-derived cannabinoids in diabetes and diabetic complications. The American Journal of Pathology. 2012;**180**:432-442. DOI: 10.1016/j.ajpath.2011.11.003

[37] Nam DH, Lee MH, Kim JE, et al. Blockade of cannabinoid receptor 1 improves insulin resistance, lipid metabolism, and diabetic nephropathy in db/db mice. Endocrinology. 2012;**153**:1387-1396. DOI: 10.1210/en.2011-1423

[38] Barutta F, Grimaldi S, Franco I, et al. Deficiency of cannabinoid receptor of type 2 worsens renal functional and structural abnormalities in streptozotocin-induced diabetic mice. Kidney International. 2014;**86**:979-990. DOI: 10.1038/ki.2014.165

[39] Barutta F, Grimaldi S, Gambino R, et al. Dual therapy targeting the endocannabinoid system prevents experimental diabetic nephropathy. Nephrology, Dialysis, Transplantation. 2017;**32**:1655-1665. DOI: 10.1093/ndt/gfx010

[40] Jourdan T, Szandaa G, Rosenberg AZ, et al. Overactive cannabinoid 1 receptor in podocytes drives type 2 diabetic nephropathy. Proceedings of the National Academy of Sciences of the United States of America. 2014;**111**:E5420-E5428. DOI: 10.1073/pnas.1419901111

[41] Zoja C, Locatelli M, Corna D, et al. Therapy with a selective cannabinoid receptor type 2 agonist limits albuminuria and renal injury in mice

with type 2 diabetic nephropathy. Nephron. 2016;**132**:59-69. DOI: 10.1159/000442679

[42] Lecru L, Desterke C, Grassin-Delyle S, et al. Cannabinoid receptor 1 is a major mediator of renal fibrosis. Kidney International. 2015;**88**:72-84. DOI: 10.1038/ki.2015.63

[43] Dao M, Lecru L, Vandermeersch S, et al. The cannabinoid receptor 1 is involved in renal fibrosis during chronic allograft dysfunction: Proof of concept. Journal of Cellular and Molecular Medicine. 2019;**23**:7279-7288. DOI: 10.1111/jcmm.14570

[44] Beger RD, Dunn W, Schmidt MA, et al. Metabolomics enables precision medicine: "A White Paper, Community Perspective". Metabolomics. 2016;**12**:1-15. DOI: 10.1007/s11306-016-1094-6

[45] Cui JJ, Wang LY, Tan ZR. Mass spectrometry-based personalized drug therapy. Mass Spectrometry Reviews. 2020;**00**:1-30. DOI: 10.1002/mas.21620

Section 2

Cannabinoids and Human Health

Chapter 4

Cannabis and the Brain: Friend or Foe?

Ali E. Dabiri and Ghassan S. Kassab

Abstract

Legalization of cannabis in the US and other countries highlight the need to understand the health consequences of this substance use. Research indicates that some cannabis ingredients may play beneficial role in treating various medical conditions while other ingredients may pose health risks. This review is focused on the brain and mental health effects of cannabis use. The rationale for examining cannabis use in behavioral and neural conditions is that these conditions are highly widespread in the US and account for high level of medical healthcare and associated cost. The purpose of this review is to provide an overview of the known medicinal benefits of selected cannabis cannabinoids in conditions like pediatric epilepsy, attention deficit hyperactivity disorder, autism spectrum disorder, and the known side effects or contraindications in conditions such as addiction, cognition, and psychosis. Several recommendations are made as to studies that will help further understanding the increasing role of cannabis in neuropsychiatric health and disease.

Keywords: cognitive, marijuana, synthetic cannabinoids, illicit substance, addiction

1. Introduction

Legalization of cannabis in the US and other countries in conjunction with increases in various methods of consumption make it vital to understand the associated health consequences. The global legal cannabis market size is expected to reach $84B by the end of 2028, according to a report by Grand View Research [1]. The cannabis market is expected to expand at a compound annual growth rate (CAGR) of 14% from 2021 to 2028 according to the report. *Gallup* poll indicates that Americans support for legalizing marijuana has been around 66% in 2018, which represents 30% increase between 2005 and 2018 [2]. In a 2019 *Gallup* poll, 13% of the US adults reported smoking cannabis, a percentage which was almost double that reported 3 years earlier [3]. About 43% of adults in the US reported having tried cannabis in 2019, 44% in 2018, 38% in 2013, and 4% in 1969 [3].

The first evidence of cannabis medicinal effects dates to Chinese medicine in the first to second century B.C. [4]. The detrimental effects of cannabis on mental health were first reported by the physician Iban Beitar between the twelfth and the thirteenth century [5]. Later in 1845, the French psychiatrist Jacque-Joseph Moreau described such effects as acute psychotic reactions that could last a few hours up to a week. He identified that the reaction was dose-dependent, and its main characteristics were illusions, hallucinations, delusions, confusion, and restlessness; and potential disorientation and loss of consciousness [6]. Such evidence suggested a potential role of cannabis in the pathophysiology of psychosis and other mental disorders, as later confirmed by studies performed over the last 50 years [7–9]. Legalization of medical and recreational cannabis has incentivized consumer to develop novel forms of cannabis consumption. The methods have been described in a recent authors' publication [10].

Here, we provide an overview of the known medicinal benefits of selected cannabis cannabinoids, the known side effects or contraindications and point out the many unknowns of cannabis use on the brain. We propose new cannabis research to answer questions as to why cannabis may be both a friend and a foe and uncover additional medicinal benefits and identify the health hazards with focus on brain and mental health.

1.1 National academies of science report

A committee on the Health Effects of cannabis consumption was formed at the National Academies of Science (NAS), Engineering and Medicine to extensively review the scientific literature and identify the research gaps. The committee formed by 16 experts in the areas of cannabis addiction, oncology, cardiology, neurodevelopment, respiratory disease, pediatric and adolescent health, immunology, toxicology, preclinical research, epidemiology, systematic review, and public health. Given the vast amount of scientific literature on cannabis, the committee decided to use published systematic reviews (since 2011) and high-quality primary research for 11 areas including brain and mental health conditions. The report was published in January 2017 [11]. The NAS committee summarized the effect of cannabis on brain and mental health literature published since 1999 [11]. The limitations of the reviewed studies included a lack of data on different methods of cannabis consumption [e.g., smoke, edible, etc.], inadequate dose information, little information on potential additives or contaminants, and lack of adequate data on total lifetime duration/dose of cannabis consumption [11]. The evidence committee found are summarized in the report [11].

2. Mechanism of action for cannabis

A large literature exists on the effects of cannabis (plant-based cannabinoids), with many of the earlier studies conducted in human subjects [12]. Recently, research on plant-based cannabinoids has been stimulated by the recognition that specific receptors exist in the brain that recognize cannabinoids, and by the discovery of a series of endogenous cannabinoids which are made in the body that act as ligands for these receptors [13]. The endocannabinoid system consists of the endogenous cannabinoids, cannabinoids receptors and the enzymes that synthesize and degrade cannabinoids. Many of the effects of cannabinoids and endocannabinoids are mediated by two G protein-coupled receptors (GPCRs), CB_1 and CB_2, although additional receptors may be involved [14]. CB_1 receptors are present in extremely high levels in several brain regions and in lower amounts in a more widespread distribution. These receptors mediate many of the psychoactive effects of cannabinoids. All these compounds act as agonists at the CB1 cannabinoid receptor [15], which is the only one known to be expressed in the brain. A second cannabinoid receptor, CB2, is expressed only in peripheral tissues, principally in the immune system [16–18]. Both CB_1 and

CB_2 coupled primarily to inhibitory G proteins and are subject to the same pharmacological influences as other GPCRs. Thus, partial agonism, functional selectivity and inverse agonism all play important roles in determining the cellular response to specific cannabinoid receptor ligands. These receptors are crucial to utilizing the active components in cannabis that influence homeostasis. Various cannabinoids have diverse effects on the receptors, functioning as agonists, antagonists, or partial antagonists, as well as affecting the vanilloid receptor [14]. The identification of cannabinoid receptors grew out of a desire to understand the psychoactive effects of Δ^9-tetrahydrocannabinol (THC), the principal psychoactive component of cannabis [18]. THC is the main activator of CB1 through allosteric modulators, which can potentially allow the therapeutic effects of THC without the intoxicating effects [18]. CNR1 gene produces the CB1 protein [19]. Since each individual carries a different version of the CNR1 gene, many people have a different experience with the use of compounds like THC and CBD [19]. THC and the synthetic cannabinoids also act to some extent as agonists at the CB2 receptor. Both cannabinoid receptors are members of the G-protein coupled class, and their activation is linked to inhibition of adenylate cyclase activity [20].

Smoking remains the most efficient means of using the drug and the users can adjust the dose by adjusting the frequency and depth of inhalation [21]. THC can also be taken orally in fat-containing foods with a delay in absorption [21]. Several man-made synthetic cannabinoids are also available [16].

3. Rationale for studies of cannabis effect on brain and mental health

Although cannabis use may impact numerous organ systems (cardiovascular, pulmonary, skeletal, etc.), we focus on the brain and mental health. There has recently been widespread interest in the relationship between cannabis use and psychosis, with over 100 papers addressing this topic each year since 2012, compared to fewer than 10 per year during the 1990s [22]. This intense interest is likely due to increasing approval within the USA of medicinal marijuana laws. Interest in this area is expected to continue to rise as cannabis becomes legally available to adults for recreational purposes. The concern is that more widespread cannabis use might increase the risk of schizophrenia [22]. Research studies indicated that heavy daily cannabis use across protracted periods exerts harmful effects on brain tissue and mental health [23]. Significant evidence exists that prenatal, perinatal, and adolescent cannabis exposure can induce a wide array of brain and behavioral alterations in adulthood [24].

4. Benefits associated with cannabis

Preliminary studies of medical marijuana suggest a variety of benefits, including improvement of chronic pain, inflammation, spasticity, and other conditions commonly seen in physical therapy practice [25]. There have been many clinical trials in a variety of conditions, including the neuropathic pain, schizophrenia, bipolar disorder, major depressive disorder, sleep deprivation and Tourette syndrome [25].

Although evidence suggests that heavy, recreational cannabis consumption is linked to cognitive deficits and potentially undesirable neural changes as outlined below, findings from studies of recreational cannabis consumption may not be applicable to medical marijuana [26]. One study examined whether patients receiving medical marijuana would exhibit improvement in cognitive functioning [27]. Further studies are warranted to clarify the specific neural and cognitive impact of medical marijuana use and how it compares to recreational use.

Investigators have evaluated the role of cannabinoids for neuroprotective role in injured brain with positive effect in acute neuronal injury [28–31]. Human clinical trials are needed to validate these outcomes and to understand the underlying mechanism involved in brain injury with use of cannabinoids.

The US Food and Drug Administration (FDA) has approved Dronabinol, the generic name for synthetic THC, is marketed under the trade name of Marinol® and is clinically indicated to counteract the nausea and vomiting associated with chemotherapy and to stimulate appetite in AIDS patients affected by wasting syndrome. A synthetic analog of THC, nabilone (Cesamet®), is prescribed for similar indications. Both dronabinol and nabilone are given orally and have a slow onset of action. In July 2016, the FDA approved Syndros®, a liquid formulation of dronabinol, for the treatment of patients experiencing chemotherapy-induced nausea and vomiting who have not responded to conventional therapies. The agent is also indicated for treating anorexia associated with weight loss in patients with AIDS. Nabiximols (Sativex®) is a combination drug standardized in composition, formulation, and dose. The principal active cannabinoid components of Sativex are the cannabinoids: tetrahydrocannabinol (THC) and cannabidiol (CBD) which was approved by UK in 2010 [32]. Nabiximols is administered as an oromucosal spray and is indicated in the symptomatic relief of multiple sclerosis [32]. Each spray delivers a dose of 2.7 mg THC and 2.5 mg CBD [32]. As of 2018, nabiximols has been launched in several countries. There are other promising applications for CBD like smoking cessation [33], drug withdrawal treatment [34], treating seizures and epilepsy [35], anxiety treatment [36], reducing some of the effects of Alzheimer's [37], and antipsychotic effects on patients with schizophrenia [38].

4.1 Pediatric epilepsy

There is significant need for safe and effective treatment of intractable childhood epilepsy, especially in cases of devastating epileptic encephalopathies, such as infantile spasms, Lennox-Gastaut syndrome [39] and Dravet syndrome [40]. Despite limited preclinical data and a lack of well-designed clinical trials, CBD, and CBD-enriched whole cannabis plant extracts, have generated excitement as potential treatments for epilepsy [41]. Following anecdotal reports of potential efficacy from parents who have administered these products to their children [42, 43], clinical trials of multiple preparations of CBD were undertaken [43–45]. The results showed strong efficacy for treatment of Lennox-Gastaut syndrome [46], Dravet syndrome [46], and highly-treatment resistant epilepsy in children and young adults [45] and confirmed reports from open-label studies [47]. Among patients with Dravet syndrome, CBD treatment resulted in a greater reduction in convulsive-seizure frequency than placebo but was associated with higher rates of adverse events [48]. The adverse effect are a risk of liver damage, lethargy, and possibly depression and thoughts of suicide from patient information leaflet, but these are also true of other treatments for epilepsy. FDA approved Epidiolex® (brand name), a purified CBD-based oral solution based on collected evidence, for the treatment of Lennox-Gastaut syndrome and Dravet syndrome in June 2018. Epidiolex® has been assigned to Schedule V of the Controlled Substances Act. Longitudinal studies are required to provide further clarification of the effects of this product in the population of interest, especially with respect to the young developing brains.

4.2 Attention deficit hyperactivity disorder (ADHD)

There are some non-scientific evidence that support the use of cannabis to treat ADHD for children and adolescents [49]. Functional Magnetic Resonance Imaging (fMRI) was employed to investigate the relation between ADHD diagnosis and cannabis consumption in young adults [50]. No impact on behavioral response inhibition on a Go/No-Go task (the Go/No-Go task is a computerized test used to assess inhibitory control, a cognitive process that enables humans to rapidly cancel motor activity even after its initiation) was observed but did find that cannabis consumption was associated with increased signal in the hippocampus and cerebellum during the fMRI only in cannabis-using control subjects, but not in cannabis-using ADHD participants [50]. This may reflect a delayed maturation trajectory in ADHD participants according to the authors and suggested further studies related to hippocampal and cerebellar function to gain more information into how this circuitry is changed by ADHD and cannabis consumption. One of the important long-term implications of a childhood diagnosis of ADHD is an increased risk for substance use, abuse, or dependence in adolescence and adulthood [51]. Longitudinal study was designed to address this research gap by recruiting a sample of 75 individuals aged 21–25 years with and without a childhood diagnosis of ADHD, who were either frequent users or non-users of cannabis. These participants were followed since age 7–9.9 [51]. The results indicated that cannabis consumption did not exacerbate ADHD-related symptoms and larger samples study was proposed. Students (n = 1738) completed an online survey containing measures of ADHD symptoms, cannabis use, perceived effects of cannabis on ADHD symptoms and medication side effects, as well as executive dysfunction [52]. They reported that cannabis has acute beneficial effects on several symptoms of ADHD (e.g., hyperactivity, impulsivity). They also perceived cannabis to improve most of their medication side effects (e.g., irritability, anxiety). Cannabis use frequency was a significant moderator of the associations between symptom severity and executive dysfunction. Results suggest people with ADHD may be using cannabis to self-medicate for many of their symptoms and medication side effects and that more frequent use may mitigate ADHD-related executive dysfunction [52].

4.3 Autism spectrum disorder (ASD)

Autism spectrum disorder (ASD) defines a group of neurodevelopmental disorders whose symptoms include impaired communication and social interaction with restricted or repetitive motor movements, frequently associated with general cognitive deficits. The endocannabinoid system is often affected in ASD patients with comorbidities, such as seizures, anxiety, cognitive impairments, and sleep disturbances [53]. There is increasing interest in cannabinoids, especially CBD as add-on treatment for the core symptoms and comorbidities of ASD. In a preclinical study that tested the efficacy of CBD in a mouse model for Dravet syndrome, CBD reduced both seizures and ASD behaviors [54]. They found that when mice were administered CBD 1 hour before induced seizures, the seizures were shorter and less severe than in the mice who did not receive CBD. The authors also found that CBD improved inhibitory neuron function, and this action could be replicated by a GPR55 antagonist, suggesting another potential therapeutic option. Presently no clinical studies have examined the effects of any cannabinoid on epilepsy reduction specifically in ASD patients. Further preclinical and clinical studies are needed to investigate the pros and cons of CBD and other cannabinoids in ASD before they are established as treatment for symptoms and co-morbidities.

5. Problems associated with cannabis

5.1 Cognition

Although cannabis and cannabinoid-based products are increasingly being accepted worldwide, there is currently limited understanding of the effect of the various cannabinoid compounds on the brain. Exogenous cannabinoids interact with the endogenous cannabinoid system that underpins vital functions in the brain to perturb key brain and cognitive function. Chye et al. [55] reviewed existing brain imaging evidence related to cannabis consumption and its major cannabinoids (THC, CBD etc.) including synthetic cannabinoid. They concluded that neuroimaging research has been limited to observational studies of cannabis users, not considering the specific role of the various cannabinoids.

Research to date has suggested that cannabis consumption leads to cognitive impairments [56] classified as acute and chronic cognition. There is strong evidence that acute administration of cannabis adversely affects executive function. Impaired performance of occasional, moderate, and heavy users was documented in some, but not all studies, on functions like reasoning, decision-making, and problem solving [57–65]. As an example, double blind experiment on 35 male mild cannabis users showed that THC administration may be a useful pharmacological cannabinoid model for psychotic effects in healthy volunteers [57]. It was found that high potency marijuana (13% THC) consistently impairs executive function and motor control in contrast with low potency marijuana (4% THC) [60]. Use of higher doses of THC in controlled experiments may offer a reliable indication of THC induced impairment as compared to lower doses of THC that have traditionally been used in performance studies [60]. Cannabis consumption has been associated with increased risk of becoming involved in traffic accidents. Ramaekers et al. [61] designed a study to investigate performance impairment as a function of THC in serum. The results indicated that serum THC concentrations between 2 and 5 ng/ml establish the lower and upper range of a THC limit for impairment.

The effects of marijuana consumption on women's cognition have been studied [64]. Anderson et al. examined sex differences in the acute effects of marijuana on cognition in 70 (35 male and 35 female) occasional users of marijuana [64]. The tasks chosen to study were divided attention, cognitive flexibility, time estimation, and visuospatial processing affected by sex and/or marijuana. The results indicated that acute marijuana use impaired performance on divided attention, time estimation, and cognitive flexibility. Although there did not appear to be sex differences in marijuana's effects on cognition, but women requested to discontinue the smoking session more often than men that led to unconclusive results.

Performance impairment during THC intoxication has been described in heavy users of cannabis [64]. Twenty-four subjects participated in a double-blind, placebo controlled, two-way mixed model design. Both groups received single doses of THC placebo and 500 μg/kg THC by smoking. Performance tests were conducted at regular intervals between 0 and 8 hrs after smoking and included measures of perceptual motor control (critical tracking task), dual task processing (divided attention task), motor inhibition (stop signal task) and cognition (Tower of London). THC significantly impaired performance of occasional cannabis users on critical tracking task, divided attention task, and the stop signal task. THC did not affect the performance of heavy cannabis users except in the stop signal task; i.e., stop reaction time increased, particularly at high THC concentrations. The comparisons of overall performance in occasional and heavy users did not reveal any persistent performance differences due to residual THC in heavy users. These data suggest that cannabis consumption history strongly determines the behavioral response to single doses of THC.

A large body evidence points to cognitive impairment after chronic, heavy cannabis consumption [66–68], lasting beyond the acute effects. There is also substantial evidence with negative findings in cannabis users [69–71]. Consistency in experimental design remains a challenging aspect of studying the long-term effects of chronic cannabis consumption on cognition [72].

Memory has been the cognitive domain most consistently impaired, with verbal learning [67, 73, 74]. In chronic users, impairments in memory and attention deteriorates with increasing years of cannabis use [68, 75–77]. Contrary to these findings, recent studies have shown that THC can promote neurogenesis, restore memory, and prevent neurodegenerative processes and cognitive decline in animal models of Alzheimer's disease [78–80]. Literature search indicates [81] that CBD improves cognition in multiple preclinical models of cognitive impairment, including models of neuropsychiatric [schizophrenia], neurodegenerative (Alzheimer's disease), neuroinflammatory (meningitis, sepsis, and cerebral malaria) and neurological disorders (hepatic encephalopathy and brain ischemia). There is only one clinical investigation into the effects of CBD on cognition in schizophrenia patients, with negative results for the Stroop test [81]. The efficacy of CBD to improve cognition in schizophrenia cannot be explained due to lack of clinical evidence. Further investigation into its efficacy in schizophrenia is justified given the ability of CBD to restore cognition in multiple impairment studies.

Studies performed on effect of cannabis on young users and showed that regular consumption during the adolescent may produce lasting adverse effects on cognitive and IQ [75, 82–83]. On the other hand, another group found little evidence that cannabis use was related to impaired cognitive performance and hypothesized that family background may explain the lower cognitive function often reported in cannabis users [84]. Another study found no relation between adolescent cannabis consumption and educational achievement [85]. It is not clear, however, whether impairment will emerge later in life. Cyrus et al. [86] reviewed the literature on the relationship between adolescent cognitive function and academic performance with cannabis consumption. The conclusion was that frequency and quantity of cannabis consumption were related with decreased functional connectivity of the brain, poorer executive control and academic performance. Factors such as minimal parental monitoring, peer cannabis consumption, social isolation, and race/ethnicity were positively correlated with more frequent adolescent use of cannabis. Interventions to prevent early initiation of cannabis use that can lead to chronic use in youth who may be more at risk was recommended.

There have been studies of the degree of cognitive function recovery with abstinence. In a study of adolescents (16–25 years of age), improvements were found in verbal memory in the first week of abstinence whose abstinence was monitored for 1 month following regular consumption [87]. Cross-sectional studies indicate improvement on attention and verbal memory but not on other cognitive domains for adolescents abstinent for 4–5 weeks [88, 89]. Further research to monitor cognitive performance improvement during prolonged periods of abstinence from chronic cannabis use are recommended to address these questions including the neural mechanisms.

The lack of assurance about the effects of cannabis consumption on cognition may be due to composition of cannabis [90]. One study showed greater memory impairment as well as signs of depression and anxiety associated with using cannabis of higher THC content compared to cannabis containing lower THC and higher levels of CBD [76]. These studies should be repeated with known THC contents to evaluate mental behavior.

A review was conducted to study the long-standing consequences regarding regular cannabis use on cognition, brain structure, and function in adults [91]. The review suggested that the neuropsychological studies provided evidence for mild cognitive deficits at least 7 days after heavy cannabis consumption. The fMRI studies showed growing evidence of abnormalities in hippocampus volume and gray matter density of cannabis users relative to controls; however, morphological changes in other brain regions were more controversial. The fMRI studies suggested an altered pattern of brain activity associated with cannabis consumption. It should be noted that there are several limitations for study comparison and substantial heterogeneity in the findings [91]. The morphological alterations could ultimately affect brain organization and function, but the associated time course for neuronal recovery as well as the real impact on cognitive functioning remain unknown. The application of fMRI is beginning to advance the understanding of the neural mechanisms associated with the cognitive consequences observed in cannabis users to establish relationship between cannabis consumption, brain function and cognitive output. Factors to be included are age of onset, mode of consumption, frequency and extent of consumption, recovery of function with abstinence with different compositions of the cannabis product. Changes in brain activity may be an early indicator of long-term consequences before cognitive deficits can be measured [56]. Application of fMRI is also important for the adolescent brain reorganization study after prolonged usage and whether these changes reverses during adulthood after abstinence.

Eadie et al. [92] determined the duration of acute neurocognitive impairment associated with medical cannabis consumption, and to identify differences between medical cannabis patients and recreational consumers. It resulted in evidence that cognitive performance in medical cannabis patients declined after THC consumption, with steady resolution of impairment in the hours following THC consumption. The degree of impairment is predominantly dose-dependent where higher doses of THC were generally more impairing than the lower doses. There was no difference on any neurocognitive test between placebo and the active THC groups at 4-hrs of recovery, irrespective of the THC dose inhaled, although the duration of neurocognitive impairment varied between studies, partly due the differences in design of experiments. More research is needed to directly relate levels of cognitive impairment to THC levels in the patients' plasma employing fMRI.

5.2 Addiction

Zehra et al. [93] reviewed the acute and long-term addiction effects of cannabis users. Cannabis use disorder (CUD) appears to correlate with the general patterns of changes described in the Koob and Volkow [94] addiction model. Previous preclinical and clinical studies seem to indicate that features of the three stages of drug addiction described by Koob and Volkow [94] are also prevalent in cannabis addiction. The model describes most drugs of abuse result in the hyperactivation of the mesocorticolimbic pathway in the binge-intoxication stage of addiction. This hyperactivation seems to be present in cannabis addiction but to a lower extent [93].

The stimulant-induced dopamine reactivity has been associated with negative emotionality, an important characteristic of withdrawal/negative affect stage explained by Koob and Volkow [94]. With the addition of withdrawal as a symptom of CUD, it is perceived that cannabis addiction development parallels addiction to other drugs of abuse. Additionally, Spechler et al. [95] found that chronic cannabis consumption has been associated with affect dysregulation that may involve changes in amygdala functioning. Cuttler et al. [96] reported that cannabis seems to disrupt hypothalamic–pituitary–adrenal (HPA) axis function as with other drugs of abuse, another key neuroadaptation of the withdrawal/negative affect stage.

Norberg et al. [97] reported that chronic cannabis consumption is also associated with the presence of cannabis cue-induced craving after abstinence, a feature of the preoccupation/anticipation stage of the Koob and Volkow framework [94]. They hypothesize that the presence of cannabis cue-induced craving seems to be related to the loss of executive control over excessive salience for cannabis. They additionally found that chronic cannabis consumption has been related to impaired memory and IQ, resulting in changes in executive functioning after chronic cannabis use.

It is imperative to investigate if there are other features of the addiction framework proposed by Koob and Volkow [94] in cannabis addiction through longitudinal studies to address behavioral and mood changes (such as changes in IQ or the presence of a mood disorder). This study should also include the synthesized cannabis due to its high potency. The relationship of addiction with the effect of THC use on neurons and microglia should also be instigated. Melis et al. [98] research result indicates that chronic THC exposure in animals seems to activate microglia and produce neuroinflammation that may underlie some of the cognitive deficits associated with CUD. Kolb et al. [99] studied changes in neuron and glia morphology after chronic cannabis exposure and concluded that it may contribute to the persistent cognitive and behavioral deficits related to CUD. Future research should investigate whether chronic THC exposure in animals and humans is related to changes in various cell types in the brain that contribute to cannabis addiction through neuroinflammation.

Combined consumption of cannabis and alcohol has increased in recent years, and it is well established that individuals who use both alcohol and cannabis are at increased risk for substance-related harms relative to individuals who use only one substance [100]. The studies provide evidence that combined consumption of alcohol and cannabis is associated with unique characteristics and psychological processes relative to single-substance use. Research in this area must continue considering recent trend toward increasingly liberal cannabis policies in the U.S. and other countries.

5.3 Psychosis

There has recently been widespread interest in the relationship between cannabis consumption and psychosis, with over 100 publications addressing this topic each year since 2012, compared to fewer than 10 per year during the 1990s [22]. This intense interest is likely due to increasing approval within the USA of medicinal marijuana laws. Cannabis consumption has seen a large increase in its licit production, growing from 1.4 tons in 2000 to 211 tons by 2016, due to the increasing implementation of medicinal programs with cannabis-related medicinal products for a wide range of neuropsychiatric conditions.

Yücel et al. [23] studied whether long-term heavy cannabis use is associated with gross anatomical abnormalities in 2 cannabinoid receptor–rich regions of the brain, the hippocampus, and the amygdala. They carefully selected 15 long-term (>10 years) and heavy (>5 joints daily) cannabis-using men (mean age, 39.8 years; mean duration of regular use, 19.7 years) with no history of polydrug abuse or neurologic/mental disorder and 16 matched non using control subjects (mean age, 36.4 years). The results indicated that cannabis users had bilaterally reduced hippocampal and amygdala volumes, with a relatively and significantly greater magnitude of reduction in the former (12.0% vs. 7.1%). Left hemisphere hippocampal volume was inversely associated with cumulative exposure to cannabis during the previous 10 years and reduced positive psychotic symptoms. Positive symptom scores were also associated with cumulative exposure to cannabis. Although cannabis users performed significantly worse than controls on verbal learning, this did not correlate with regional brain volumes in either group. These results provide new evidence of exposure-related structural abnormalities in the hippocampus and amygdala in long-term heavy cannabis users with similar findings in the animal literature. The findings indicated that heavy daily cannabis consumption for long periods exerts harmful effects on brain tissue and mental health.

Hurd et al. [24] reviewed several investigations and concluded that strong evidence exists that prenatal, perinatal, and adolescent cannabis exposure can cause a series of brain and behavioral changes in adulthood. This happens through interfering with multiple neurobiological systems in brain regions involved in psychotic/affective disorders. Adolescent cannabis consumption is associated with an increased risk for psychosis later in life [101]. Whether such risk truly results in psychiatric, and substance use disorders will depend on various factors, such as genetics, age, frequency of use, concurrent use of other substances and sex, that will be better understood as research continues to expand. They recommended that policy makers need to apply the existing data to educate the public about the potential health risk and the long-term effects on adult mental health.

THC or other cannabinoid agonists all suffer from the problem of a narrow therapeutic window between the desired clinical benefits and the unwanted psychic side-effects. It is possible that the pharmacological manipulation of the endocannabinoid system by drugs that inhibited the inactivation of the endocannabinoids, may offer a safer and more subtle approach to cannabis-based medicines in the future [102].

Empirical evidence suggests that cannabis consumption is associated with both CUD and comorbid psychiatric illness, which is not perceived to be the case by the US general population. On the other hand, there is mixed evidence regarding the role of cannabis in the prognosis of a co-occurring disorder across all categories of psychiatric disorders [103]. It can be concluded that longitudinal effort needs to be performed to expand on the existing body of literature to better understand the acute and long-term effects of cannabis on comorbid psychiatric illness.

6. Unknowns associated with cannabis consumption/synthetic illicit drugs

It is imperative that cannabis legalization which will likely increase cannabis use, does not cause significant adverse effect like tobacco smoking. This topic was discussed in previous authors' publication [10]. It is recommended that research be conducted on the long- and short-term health effects of exposure to second-hand marijuana smoking to confirm possible adverse effect on brain and mental health. The large market of cannabis has given rise to numerous potentially hazardous natural contaminants being reported in crude cannabis and preparations. This topic also was discussed in previous authors' publication [10]. These drugs have detrimental effects on the brain and primarily affect the central nervous system. Understanding the mechanism of brain alteration due to synthetic drug abuse can help with early detection, diagnosis, and prognosis of brain tissue damage in the clinical setting. Furthermore, these drugs sometimes have severe, life-threatening adverse effects on the human body. A few structural MRI studies have been conducted in synthetic drug abusers to reveal the effects of these drugs on the brain [104] to offer treatment options for various class of synthetic drugs.

7. Conclusions and recommendations

Legalization of cannabis in the US and other counties in conjunction with increase in various methods of consumption makes it vital to understand the associated health consequences. There are indications to suggest that many compounds found in cannabis have potential therapeutic benefit, either alone or in combination with other cannabinoid or terpene compounds [105].

Further pre-clinical and clinical studies are needed to examine the pros and cons of CBD and other cannabinoids in ASD, ADHD, and pediatric epilepsy before they are established as treatment. Further research is needed to better understand the acute and long-term effects of cannabis on comorbid psychiatric illness. Further application of fMRI is recommended to understand the adolescent brain reorganization after prolonged usage and whether these changes reverses during adulthood after abstinence. Future studies should investigate whether chronic THC exposure is linked to changes in various cell types in the brain that contribute to cannabis addiction. Cannabis addiction findings indicate that neurobiological changes in CUD seem to parallel those in other addictions. Further research is necessary in view of recent increase in cannabis consumption. Increasing number of new research concluded that significant evidence exists that prenatal, perinatal, and adolescent cannabis exposure can induce a wide array of brain and behavioral alterations in adulthood. New research is warranted to better understand the risk involved as function of various parameters such as genetics and sex. Research that identifies any potential effects of cannabis secondhand smoking (CSHS) on potential changes in cognitive function is important if consumption in public access areas is being considered.

Present research studies on how cannabis exposure can impact brain and mental health are beginning to inform public policy decision makers, including acceptable age of consumption, dose limits and directions for use. Nonetheless, additional investigation is required to fully understand the impact of cannabis on the cognition, especially for CBD where there may be various confounding biological variables unique to individual medical conditions. The impact of cannabis on the still-developing adolescent brain deserves special attention. While recreational use among adolescents and early onset users is relatively well studied, some areas remain understudied and need data to inform changing public policy. For example, additional effort is required to fully understand the impact of moderate cannabis consumption, short- and long-term consequences of using high-potency cannabis and new delivery methods, effects of cannabis consumption in older adults, and the efficacy and safety of existing and future products. Field-wide difficulties in quantification, methods of measuring cognitive constructs, and the influence of subacute effects seriously hamper the road ahead and require attention now. Multidisciplinary collaboration and investment in studies that solve these problems should be prioritized.

Although existing data suggest that there are findings regarding the chronic and acute effects of cannabis on brain activity, but refinements may help answer questions regarding potential differences between those persons who become dependent on cannabis versus those who use cannabis recreationally, potential residual effects of chronic use, consequences of earlier age of exposure to cannabis, acute and chronic effects on task performance, and possible neurobiological similarities between comorbid psychiatric disorders and cannabis consumption. Future effort using specific diagnostic criteria, and combining neurocognitive testing to functional imaging, may help address questions including the basis of any residual cognitive deficits from cannabis consumption and any potential factors differentiating cannabis-dependent subjects from cannabis users.

The mechanisms that underlie associations between cannabis consumption with psychiatric illness and cognitive impairment are still not well understood, although epidemiological and clinical studies have consistently established this relationship. It is well established that exposure during adolescence is a period of high risk, resulting in more severe and persistent adverse effects than exposure during adulthood. It is plausible that prolonged consumption during adolescence results in a disruption in the normative neuro-maturational processes. Eventually, this could result in long lasting changes to brain structure and function that underlie many of the adverse cognitive and emotional outcomes associated with heavy consumption. Spreading awareness regarding the potential risk of cognitive disturbance in adolescent cannabis users and screening them at an earlier age for potential risk factors of future cognitive damages should be encouraged among healthcare providers. Clearly, further investigation is needed to study the cognitive effects of synthetic cannabinoids to inform the public policy to curb the spread of synthetic cannabinoids and to keep the risk/benefit ratio of the medicinal consumption of cannabis as low as possible. Furthermore, the role of medicinal cannabis including benefits and potential risks with regards to brain management need to be studied in randomized experiments.

The emerging research on cannabis and alcohol co-use and associated outcomes has the potential to inform intervention efforts. As research on the combined use of cannabis and alcohol continues to evolve, next step would be to develop a program that target co-use as a specific high-risk behavior. We hope that new studies will help further understanding of the increasing role of cannabis in neuropsychiatric health and disease. We also hope to soon witness advances in the field of cannabis-related pharmacological treatments.

Finally, it is important to distinguish between scientifically studied and FDA approved cannabis benefits as opposed to potential benefits for indications not rigorously studied, e.g., attention deficit hyperactivity disorder. Conversely, there are situations where rigorous controlled clinical studies have been successfully completed to establish the scientific credibility of cannabis for certain indications but has not yet completed regulatory approval. It is essential that both scientific rigor and regulatory approval support a specific therapy for cannabis.

Conflict of interest

The authors have no financial conflicts of interest to declare.

Statements and declarations

Consent for publication: The authors have given their consent for publication.
Funding: The work is funded by 3DTholdings, LLC.

Author details

Ali E. Dabiri[1*] and Ghassan S. Kassab[2]

1 3DT Holdings, San Diego, CA, USA

2 California Medical Innovation Institute, San Diego, CA, USA

*Address all correspondence to: adabiri@3dtholdings.com

References

[1] Available from: https://www.grandviewresearch.com/press-release/global-legal-marijuana-market

[2] Available from: https://news.gallup.com/poll/267698/support-legal-marijuana-steady-past-year.aspx

[3] Available from: https://news.gallup.com/poll/194195/adults-say-smoke-marijuana.aspx

[4] Brand EJ, Zhao Z. Cannabis in Chinese medicine: Are some traditional indications referenced in ancient literature related to cannabinoids? Frontiers in Pharmacology. 2017;**8**. Article ID: 108

[5] Dhunjibhoy JE. A brief resume of the types of insanity commonly met with in India with a full description of "Indian hemp insanity" peculiar to the country. The Journal of Mental Science. 1930;**76**:254-264

[6] Moreau JJ. Du Hachisch et de L'aliénation Mentale: Études Psychologiques. Fortin Masson: Paris, France; 1845

[7] Colizzi M, Bhattacharyya S. Is there sufficient evidence that cannabis use is a risk factor for psychosis? In: Thompson AD, Broome MR, editors. Risk Factors for Psychosis: Paradigms, Mechanisms, and Prevention. Cambridge, MA, USA: Academic Press; 2020. pp. 305-331

[8] Colizzi M, Ruggeri M, Bhattacharyya S. Unraveling the intoxicating and therapeutic effects of cannabis ingredients on psychosis and cognition. Frontiers in Psychology. 2020;**11**:833

[9] Colizzi M, Bhattacharyya S. Cannabis: Neuropsychiatry and its effects on brain and behavior. Brain Sciences. 2020;**10**(11):834

[10] Dabiri AE, Kassab GS. Medical Cannabis and Cannabinoids. 2021;**4**: 75-85. DOI: 10.1159/000519775

[11] National Academy of Sciences, Engineering, and Medicine. The Health Effects of Cannabis and Cannabinoids: The Current State of Evidence and Recommendations for Research. Washington, DC: The National Academies Press; 2017. DOI: 10.17226/24625

[12] Hollister LE. Health aspects of cannabis. Pharmacological Reviews. 1986;**38**:1-20

[13] Iversen L. Cannabis and the brain. Brain. 2003;**126**:1252-1270

[14] Mackie K. Cannabinoid receptors: Where they are and what they do. Journal of Neuroendocrinology. 2008;**20**(s1):10-14

[15] Matsuda LA, Lolait SJ, Brownstein MJ, Young AC, Bonner TI. Structure of a cannabinoid receptor and functional expression of the cloned cDNA. Nature. 1990;**346**(6284):561-564. DOI: 10.1038/346561a0

[16] Pertwee RG. Pharmacology of cannabinoid receptor ligands. Current Medicinal Chemistry. 1999;**6**:635-664

[17] Munro S, Thomas KL, Abu-Shaar M. Molecular characterization of a peripheral receptor for cannabinoids. Nature. 1993;**365**:61-65

[18] Felder CC, Glass M. Cannabinoid receptors and their endogenous agonists. Annual Review of Pharmacology and Toxicology. 1998;**38**:179-200

[19] Tao R, Li C, Jaffe AE, Shin JH, Deep-Soboslay A, Yamin R'e, et al. Cannabinoid receptor CNR1 expression and DNA methylation in human prefrontal cortex, hippocampus and caudate in brain development and schizophrenia. Translational Psychiatry. 2020;**10**:158. DOI: 10.1038/s41398-020-0832-8

[20] Howlett AC, Johnson MR, Melvin LS, Milne GM. Nonclassical cannabinoid analgesics inhibit adenylate cyclase: Development of a cannabinoid receptor model. Molecular Pharmacology. 1988;**33**:297-302

[21] Iversen LL. The Science of Marijuana. Oxford: Oxford University Press; 2000

[22] Ksir C, Hart CL. Cannabis and psychosis: A critical overview of the relationship. Current Psychiatry Reports. 2016;**18**:12

[23] Yucel M, Solowij N, Respondek C, Whittle S, Fornito A, Pantelis C, et al. Regional brain abnormalities associated with long-term heavy cannabis use. Archives of General Psychiatry. 2008;**65**(6):694-701

[24] Hurd YL, Manzoni OJ, Pletnikov MV, Lee FS, Bhattacharyya S, Melis M. Cannabis and the developing brain: Insights into its long-lasting effects. Journal of Neuroscience. 2019;**39**(42):8250-8258

[25] Ciccone CD. Medical marijuana: Just the beginning of a long, strange trip? Physical Therapy. 2017;**97**:239-248

[26] Sagar KA, Gruber SA. Marijuana matters: Reviewing the impact of marijuana on cognition, brain structure and function, & exploring policy implications and barriers to research. International Review of Psychiatry. 2018;**30**:251-267. DOI: 10.1080/09540261.2018.1460334

[27] Gruber SA, Sagar KA, Dahlgren MK, Yao X, Levine SJ. Splendor in the grass? A pilot study assessing the impact of medical marijuana on executive function. Frontiers in Pharmacology. 2016;7:355. DOI: 10.3389/fphar.2016.00323

[28] Grundy RI. The therapeutic potential of the cannabinoids in neuroprotection. Expert Opinion on Investigational Drugs. 2002;**11**:1365-1374. DOI: 10.1517/13543784.11.10.1365

[29] Latorre JGS, Schmidt EB. Cannabis, cannabinoids, and cerebral metabolism: Potential applications in stroke and disorders of the central nervous system. Current Cardiology Reports. 2015;**17**:627. DOI: 10.1007/s11886-015-0627-3

[30] Magid L, Heymann S, Elgali M, Millis SR, Scott C, Pearson C. Role of CB2 receptor in the recovery of mice after traumatic brain injury. Journal of Neurotrauma. 2019;**36**:1836-1846. DOI: 10.1089/neu. 2018.5873

[31] Shohami E, Cohen-Yeshurun A, Magid L, Facciolo F, Rendina EA, Page C, et al. Endocannabinoids and traumatic brain injury. British Journal of Pharmacology. 2011;**163**:1402-1410. DOI: 10.1111/j.1476-5381.2011.01339. x

[32] Wikipedia, July 2022

[33] Morgan CJ, Das RK, Joye A, Curran HV, Kamboj SK. Cannabidiol reduces cigarette consumption in tobacco smokers: Preliminary findings. Addictive Behaviors. 2013;**38**(9):2433-2436

[34] Hurd YL, Yoon M, Manini AF, Hernandez S, Olmedo R, Ostman M, et al. Early phase in the development of Cannabidiol as a treatment for addiction:

Opioid relapse takes initial center stage. Neurotherapeutics. 2015;**12**(4):807-815

[35] Devinsky O, Cilio MR, Cross H, Fernandez-Ruiz J, French J, Hill C, et al. Cannabidiol: Pharmacology and potential therapeutic role in epilepsy and other neuropsychiatric disorders. Epilepsia. 2014;**55**(6):791-802

[36] Blessing EM, Steenkamp MM, Manzanares J, Marmar CR. Cannabidiol as a potential treatment for anxiety disorders. Neurotherapeutics. 2015;**12**(4):825-836

[37] Cheng D, Spiro AS, Jenner AM, Garner B, Karl T. Long-term Cannabidiol treatment prevents the development of social recognition memory deficits in Alzheimer's disease transgenic mice. Journal of Alzheimer's Disease. 2014;**42**(4):1383-1396

[38] Zuardi AW. A critical review of the antipsychotic effects of cannabidiol: 30 years of a translational investigation. Current Pharmaceutical Design. 2012;**18**(32):5131-5140

[39] Hussain S, Sankar R. Pharmacologic treatment of intractable epilepsy in children: A syndrome-based approach. Seminars in Pediatric Neurology. 2011;**18**:171-178. DOI: 10.1016/j.spen.2011.06.003

[40] Wirrell EC. Treatment of Dravet syndrome. Canadian Journal of Neurological Sciences. 2016;**43**:S13-S18

[41] Szaflarski JP, Bebin EM. Cannabis, cannabidiol, and epilepsy–from receptors to clinical response. Epilepsy & Behavior. 2014;**41**:277-282

[42] Hussain SA, Zhou R, Jacobson C, Weng J, Cheng E, Lay J, et al. Perceived efficacy of cannabidiol-enriched cannabis extracts for treatment of pediatric epilepsy: A potential role for infantile spasms and Lennox-Gastaut syndrome. Epilepsy & Behavior. 2015;**47**:138-141

[43] Sirven JI. Cannabis, cannabidiol, and epilepsies: The truth is somewhere in the middle. Epilepsy & Behavior. 2014;**41**:270-271

[44] Cilio MR, Thiele EA, Devinsky O. The case for assessing cannabidiol in epilepsy. Epilepsia. 2014;**55**:787-790

[45] Devinsky O, Marsh E, Friedman D, Thiele E, Laux L, Sullivan J, et al. Cannabidiol in patients with treatment-resistant epilepsy: An open-label interventional trial. Lancet Neurology. 2016;**15**:270-278

[46] Thiele EA, Marsh ED, French JA, Mazurkiewicz-Beldzinska M, Benbadis SR, Joshi C, et al. Cannabidiol in patients with seizures associated with Lennox-Gastaut syndrome [GWPCARE4]: A randomized, double-blind, placebo-controlled phase 3 trial. Lancet. 2018;**391**:1085-1096

[47] McCoy B, Wang L, Zak M, Al-Mehmadi S, Kabir N, Alhadid K, et al. A prospective open-label trial of a CBD/THC cannabis oil in dravet syndrome. Annals of Clinical Translational Neurology. 2018;**5**:1077-1088

[48] Devinsky O, Cross JH, Laux L, Marsh E, Miller I, Nabbout R, et al. Trial of Cannabidiol for drug-resistant seizures in the Dravet syndrome. The New England Journal of Medicine. 2017;**376**:2011-2020. DOI: 10.1056/NEJMoa1611618

[49] Mitchell JT, Sweitzer MM, Tunno AM, Kollins SH, McClernon FJ, Lidzba K. "I use weed for my ADHD": A qualitative analysis of online forum discussions on cannabis use and ADHD. PLoS One. 2016;**11**:e0156614

[50] Rasmussen J, Casey BJ, van Erp TGM, Tamm L, Epstein JN, Buss C, et al. ADHD and cannabis use in young adults examined using fMRI of a Go/NoGo task. Brain Imaging and Behavior. 2016;**10**:761-771

[51] Kelly C, Castellanos FX, Tomaselli O, Lisdahl K, Tamm L, Jernigan T, et al. Distinct effects of childhood ADHD and cannabis use on brain functional architecture in young adults. NeuroImage: Clinical. 2017;**13**:188-200

[52] Stueber A, Cuttler C. Self-reported effects of cannabis on ADHD symptoms, ADHD medication side effects, and ADHD-related executive dysfunction. Journal of Attention Disorders. 2022;**26**(6):942-955. DOI: 10.1177/10870547211050949

[53] Zamberletti E, Gabaglio M, Parolaro D. The endocannabinoid system and autism spectrum disorders: Insights from animal models. International Journal of Molecular Sciences. 2017;**18**:1916

[54] Kaplan JS, Stella N, Catterall WA, Westenbroek RE. Cannabidiol attenuates seizures and social deficits in a mouse model of Dravet syndrome. Proceedings of the National Academy of Sciences. 2017;**114**:11229-11234

[55] Chye Y, Kirkham R, Lorenzetti V, McTavish E, Solowij N, Yücel M. Cannabis, cannabinoids, and brain morphology: A review of the evidence. Biological Psychiatry: Cognitive Neuroscience and Neuroimaging. 2021;**6**(6):627-635

[56] Burggren AC, Shirazi A, Ginder N, Edythe D. London cannabis effects on brain structure, function, and cognition: Considerations for medical uses of cannabis and its derivatives. The American Journal of Drug and Alcohol Abuse. 2019;**45**(6):563-579

[57] Liem-Moolenaar M, Te Beek ET, de Kam ML, Franson KL, Kahn RS, Hijman R, et al. Central nervous system effects of haloperidol on THC in healthy male volunteers. Journal of Psychopharmacology. 2010;**24**:1697-1708. DOI: 10.1177/0269881109358200

[58] Metrik J, Kahler CW, Reynolds B, McGeary JE, Monti PM, Haney M, et al. Balanced placebo design with marijuana: Pharmacological and expectancy effects on impulsivity and risk taking. Psychopharmacology. 2012;**223**:489-499. DOI: 10.1007/s00213-012-2740-y

[59] Morrison PD, Zois V, McKeown DA, Jennaway M, Basudewa IDG, Taylor R. The acute effects of synthetic intravenous Delta9-tetrahydrocannabinol on psychosis, mood and cognitive functioning. Psychological Medicine. 2009;**39**:1607-1616. DOI: 10.1017/S0033291708004893

[60] Ramaekers JG, Kauert G, van Ruitenbeek P, Theunissen EL, Schneider E, Moeller MR. High-potency marijuana impairs executive function and inhibitory motor control. Neuropsychopharmacology. 2006;**31**:2296-2303. DOI: 10.1038/sj.npp.1301068

[61] Ramaekers JG, Moeller MR, van Ruitenbeek P, Theunissen EL, Schneider E, Kauert G. Cognition and motor control as a function of Delta9-THC concentration in serum and oral fluid: Limits of impairment. Drug and Alcohol Dependence. 2006;**85**:114-122. DOI: 10.1016/j.drugalcdep.2006.03.015

[62] Weinstein A, Brickner O, Lerman H, Greemland M, Bloch M, Lester H, et al. A study investigating the acute dose-response effects of 13 mg and 17 mg Delta 9-tetrahydrocannabinol on cognitive-motor skills, subjective and autonomic measures in regular

users of marijuana. Journal of Psychopharmacology. 2008;**22**:441-451. DOI: 10.1177/0269881108088194

[63] Anderson BM, Rizzo M, Block RI, Pearlson GD, O'Leary DS. Sex, drugs, and cognition: Effects of marijuana. Journal of Psychoactive Drugs. 2010;**42**:413-424. DOI: 10.1080/02791072.2010.10400704

[64] Ramaekers JG, Kauert G, Theunissen EL, Toennes SW, Moeller MR. Neurocognitive performance during acute THC intoxication in heavy and occasional cannabis users. Journal of Psychopharmacology. 2009;**23**:266-277. DOI: 10.1177/0269881108092393

[65] Ranganathan M, Carbuto M, Braley G, Elander J, Perry E, Pittman B, et al. Naltrexone does not attenuate the effects of intravenous Δ9-tetrahydrocannabinol in healthy humans. The International Journal of Neuropsychopharmacology. 2012;**15**:1251-1264. DOI: 10.1017/S1461145711001830

[66] Schmetzer AD. Book review: Cannabis and cognitive functioning, by Nadia Solowij. Annals of Clinical Psychiatry. 2000;**12**:254-257. DOI: 10.1023/A:1009051030174

[67] Solowij N, Battisti R. The chronic effects of cannabis on memory in humans: A review. Current Drug Abuse Reviews. 2008;**1**:81-98. DOI: 10.2174/1874473710801010081

[68] Solowij N, Babor T, Stephens R, Roffman RA. Does marijuana use cause long-term cognitive deficits? JAMA. 2002;**287**:2653-2654

[69] Fontes MA, Bolla KI, Cunha PJ, Almeida PP, Jungerman F, Laranjeira RR, et al. Cannabis use before age 15 and subsequent executive functioning. The British Journal of Psychiatry: the Journal of Mental Science. 2011;**198**:442-447. DOI: 10.1192/bjp.bp.110.077479

[70] Hester R, Nestor L, Garavan H. Impaired error awareness and anterior cingulate cortex hypoactivity in chronic cannabis users. Neuropsychopharmacology. 2009;**34**:2450-2458. DOI: 10.1038/npp.2009.67

[71] Tait RJ, Mackinnon A, Christensen H. Cannabis use and cognitive function: 8-year trajectory in a young adult cohort. Addiction. 2011;**106**:2195-2203. DOI: 10.1111/j.1360-0443.2011.03574. x

[72] Mokrysz C, Freeman TP, Commentary on Meier, et al. Smoke and mirrors-are adolescent cannabis users vulnerable to cognitive impairment? Addiction. 2018;**113**:266-267. DOI: 10.1111/add.14055

[73] Broyd SJ, van Hell HH, Beale C, Yücel M, Solowij N. Acute and chronic effects of cannabinoids on human cognition-a systematic review. Biological Psychiatry. 2016;**79**:557-567. DOI: 10.1016/j.biopsych.2015.12.002

[74] Ganzer F, Broning S, Kraft S, Sack P-M, Thomasius R. Weighing the evidence: A systematic review on long-term neurocognitive effects of cannabis use in abstinent adolescents and adults. Neuropsychology Review. 2016;**26**:186-222. DOI: 10.1007/s11065-016-9316-2

[75] Meier MH, Caspi A, Ambler A, Harrington H, Houts R, Keefe RSE, et al. Persistent cannabis users show neuropsychological decline from childhood to midlife. Proceedings of the National Academy of Sciences of the United States of America. 2012;**109**:E2657-E2664. DOI: 10.1073/pnas.1206820109

[76] Morgan CJA, Gardener C, Schafer G, Swan S, Demarchi C, Freeman TP, et al. Sub-chronic impact of cannabinoids in street cannabis on cognition, psychotic-like symptoms, and psychological well-being. Psychological Medicine. 2012;**42**:391-400. DOI: 10.1017/S0033291711001322

[77] Solowij N, Stephens RS, Roffman RA, Babor T, Kadden R, Miller M, et al. Cognitive functioning of long-term heavy cannabis users seeking treatment. JAMA. 2002;**287**:1123-1131

[78] Bilkei-Gorzo A, Albayram O, Draffehn A, et al. A chronic low dose of Δ9-tetrahydrocannabinol [THC] restores cognitive function in old mice. Nature Medicine. 2017;**23**:782-787. DOI: 10.1038/nm.4265

[79] Martín-Moreno AM, Brera B, Spuch C, Carro E, García-García L, Delgado M, et al. Prolonged oral cannabinoid administration prevents neuroinflammation, lowers β-amyloid levels and improves cognitive performance in Tg APP 2576 mice. Journal of Neuroinflammation. 2012;**9**:8. DOI: 10.1186/1742-2094-9-8

[80] Ramírez BG, Blázquez C, Gómez Del Pulgar T, Guzmán M, de Ceballos ML. Prevention of Alzheimer's disease pathology by cannabinoids: Neuroprotection mediated by blockade of microglial activation. Journal of Neuroscience: The Official Journal of the Society for Neuroscience. 2005;**25**:1904-1913

[81] Osborne AL, Solowij N, Weston-Green K. A systematic review of the effect of cannabidiol on cognitive function: Relevance to schizophrenia. Neuroscience and Biobehavioral Reviews. 2017;**72**:310-324. DOI: 10.1016/j.neubiorev.2016.11.012

[82] Levine A, Clemenza K, Rynn M, Lieberman J. Evidence for the risks and consequences of adolescent cannabis exposure. Journal of the American Academy of Child and Adolescent Psychiatry. 2017;**56**(3):214-225. DOI: 10.1016/j.jaac.2016.12.014

[83] Lisdahl KM, Wright NE, Kirchner-Medina C, Maple KE, Shollenbarger S. Considering cannabis: The effects of regular cannabis use on neurocognition in adolescents and young adults. Current Addiction Reports. 2014;**1**:144-156. DOI: 10.1007/s40429-014-0019-6

[84] Meier MH, Caspi A, Danese A, Fisher HL, Houts R, Arseneault L, et al. Associations between adolescent cannabis use and neuropsychological decline: A longitudinal co-twin control study. Addiction. 2018;**113**:257-265. DOI: 10.1111/add.v113.2

[85] Mokrysz C, Landy R, Gage SH, Munafò MR, Roiser JP, Curran HV. Are IQ and educational outcomes in teenagers related to their cannabis use? A prospective cohort study. Journal of Psychopharmacology. 2016;**30**:159-168. DOI: 10.1177/0269881115622241

[86] Cyrus E, Coudray MS, Kiplagat S, Mariano Y, Noel I, Galea JT, et al. A review investigating the relationship between cannabis use and adolescent cognitive functioning. Current Opinion in Psychology. 2021;**38**:38-48

[87] Schuster RM, Gilman J, Schoenfeld D, Evenden J, Hareli M, Ulysse C, et al. One month of cannabis abstinence in adolescents and young adults is associated with improved memory. The Journal of Clinical Psychiatry. 2018;**79**(6). DOI: 10.4088/JCP.17m11977

[88] Medina KL, Hanson KL, Schweinsburg AD, COHEN-ZION

M, NAGEL BJ, TAPERT SF. Neuropsychological functioning in adolescent marijuana users: Subtle deficits detectable after a month of abstinence. Journal of the International Neuropsychological Society. 2007;**13**:807-820. DOI: 10.1017/S1355617707071032

[89] Winward JL, Hanson KL, Tapert SF, Brown SA. Heavy alcohol use, marijuana use, and concomitant use by adolescents are associated with unique and shared cognitive decrements. Journal of the international Neuropsychological Society. 2014;**20**:784-795. DOI: 10.1017/S1355617714000666

[90] Colizzi M, Bhattacharyya S. Does cannabis composition matter? Differential effects of delta-9-tetrahydrocannabinol and Cannabidiol on human cognition. Current Addiction Reports. 2017;**4**:62-74. DOI: 10.1007/s40429-017-0142-2

[91] Nader DA, Sanchez ZM. Effects of regular cannabis use on neurocognition, brain structure, and function: A systematic review of findings in adults. The American Journal of Drug and Alcohol Abuse. 2018;**44**:4-18. DOI: 10.1080/00952990.2017.1306746

[92] Eadie L, Lo LA, Christiansen A, Brubacher JR, Barr AM, Panenka WJ, et al. Duration of neurocognitive impairment with medical cannabis use: A scoping review. Frontiers in Psychiatry. 2021. DOI: 10.3389/fpsyt.2021.638962

[93] Zehra A, Burns J, Liu CK, Manza P, Wiers CE, Volkow ND, et al. Cannabis addiction and the brain: A review. Journal of Neuroimmune Pharmacology. 2018;**13**:438-452

[94] Koob GF, Volkow ND. Neurobiology of addiction: A neurocircuitry analysis. Lancet Psychiatry. 2016;**3**:760-773

[95] Spechler PA, Orr CA, Chaarani B, Kan KJ, Mackey S, Morton A, et al. IMAGEN consortium. Cannabis use in early adolescence: Evidence of amygdala hypersensitivity to signals of threat. Developmental Cognitive Neuroscience. 2015;**16**:63-70

[96] Cuttler C, Spradlin A, Nusbaum AT, Whitney P, Hinson JM, McLaughlin RJ. Blunted stress reactivity in chronic cannabis users. Psychopharmacology. 2017;**234**:2299-2309

[97] Norberg MM, Kavanagh DJ, Olivier J, Lyras S. Craving cannabis: A meta-analysis of self-report and psychophysiological cue-reactivity studies. Addiction. 2016;**111**:1923-1934

[98] Melis M, Frau R, Kalivas PW, Spencer S, Chioma V, Zamberletti E, et al. New vistas on cannabis use disorder. Neuropharmacology. 2017;**124**:62-72. DOI: 10.1016/j.neuropharm.2017.03.033

[99] Kolb B, Li Y, Robinson T, Parker LA. THC alters morphology of neurons in medial prefrontal cortex, orbital prefrontal cortex, and nucleus accumbens and alters the ability of later experience to promote structural plasticity. Synapse. Mar 2018;**72**(3). DOI: 10.1002/syn.22020

[100] Linden-Carmichael AN, Wardell JD. Combined use of alcohol and cannabis: Introduction to the special issue. Psychology of Addictive Behaviors. 2021;**35**(6):621-627. DOI: 10.1037/adb0000772

[101] Kiburi SK, Molebatsi K, Ntlantsana V, Lynskey MT. Cannabis use in adolescence and risk of psychosis: Are there factors that moderate this relationship? A systematic review and meta-analysis. Substance Abuse. 2021;**42**(4):527-542. DOI: 10.1080/08897077.2021.1876200

[102] Hillmer A, Chawar C, Sanger S, D'Elia A, Butt M, Kapoor R, et al. Genetic basis of cannabis use: A systematic review. BMC Medical Genomics. 2021;**14**:203

[103] Hasin D, Walsh C. Cannabis use, cannabis use disorder, and comorbid psychiatric illness: A narrative review. Journal of Clinical Medicine. 2021;**10**(1):15. DOI: 10.3390/jcm10010015

[104] Creagh S, Warden D, Latif MA, Paydar A. The new classes of synthetic illicit drugs can significantly harm the brain: A neuro imaging perspective with full review of MRI findings. Clinical Radiology & Imaging Journal. 2018;**2**(1):000116

[105] Russo EB, Taming THC. Potential cannabis synergy and phytocannabinoid-terpenoid entourage effects. British Journal of Pharmacology. 2011;**163**:1344-1364

Chapter 5

Pediatric Brain on Cannabinoids: Adverse Effects of Cannabinoid Products in Children and Adolescents

Peter B. Chase

Abstract

Cannabinoids (phytocannabinoids and synthetic cannabinoids) are most often used during adolescence and given the changing norms, enhanced potency, reduced societal perceptions of risk and multitude forms of products for consumption, clinicians need to be become more cognizant of cannabinoid products and their effects. The aim of this narrative review is to briefly discuss acute toxicities and a few chronic toxicities associated with cannabinoids that clinicians are likely to treat. In addition, cannabinoid toxicokinetics and toxicodynamics as it pertains to the clinical effects will be discussed as well as the route of exposure and the clinical implications for therapeutics. Although the neurodevelopmental effects of naturally occurring endocannabinoids will be briefly mentioned, it is beyond the scope of this review to discuss in detail. Regardless, clinicians, parents and patients should be aware of the potential implications that exogenous cannabinoids (cannabis) may have in altering the normative trajectory of brain maturation in pediatric patients.

Keywords: cannabinoids, synthetic, THC, toxicity, pediatric

1. Introduction

Cannabis (*Cannabis sativa*) has been widely studied and is used for recreational, medicinal and in scientific research with its principle bioactive components being cannabinoids. The term "Cannabis" is actually the genus of the flowering plant whose well known species include *sativia*, *indica*, and *ruderalis*. When the cannabis flower bud/leaves are dried, it is referred to as marijuana [1] as long as the plant contains more than 0.3% of THC, otherwise it is referred to as hemp. Cannabis is comprised of over 100 different cannabinoids and non-cannabinoid substances and is a complex psychoactive plant that contains many cannabinoid components of unclear effects and they have commonly been neglected [2]. The four most abundant cannabinoids are Delta-9 tetrahydrocannabinol (Delta-9 THC, or THC), cannabinol

(CBN), cannabidiol (CBD), and cannabigerol (CBG) [3]. The abuse related potential of cannabis is mediated by THC, the main phytocannabinoid component thought to be responsible for the majority of the psychoactive, mood altering and reinforcing properties of cannabis.

Sativia variety has the highest percentage of THC with *indica* and *ruderalis* varieties have the higher percentages of CBD [4]. It is the ratio of THC/CBD that defines potency and its psychoactive effects. Of course, there are hybrid varieties making it even more difficult to know what the THC/CBD ratio is, and consequently the potency. Higher potency is associated with euphoric, anxiolytic and relaxing effects while lower potency is usually more sedating and similar to medical cannabis. Through the years there has been global increases in THC levels and decreases in CBD levels and both (increases in THC potency and decreases in CBD) have been implicated in causing health complications from cannabis use [5]. CBD is non intoxicating and appears to minimize some harmful effects of THC including memory impairment and psychotic symptoms. As a result, evidence appears to indicate that the potency of THC and CBD and their relative ratios are important factors in determining the level of harm an individual may experience [6].

Based on the etiology of the cannabinoids, they are generally separated into three groups: endocannabinoids, phytocannabinoids and synthetic cannabinoids. Endocannabinoids (eCB) are endogenously produced in the human body and are lipid ligands that interact with at least two "G-protein" coupled receptors (CB1 and CB2) located in the brain and peripheral nervous system. The activation of these receptors causes an inhibition of the release of neurotransmitters (acetylcholine and glutamate) and indirectly effecting many other receptors. The CB1 and CB2 receptors are located presynaptically which means that cannabinoids modulate neurotransmitter release [7]. The concern during prenatal and post birth development through the adolescent years is that exogenous cannabinoids may alter the neurodevelopment of the brain since evidence points to CB1 receptors being more prevalent during developing years than in the adult [8]. Phytocannabinoids are naturally occurring cannabinoids found in the cannabis plant with the four most abundant cannabinoids already mentioned above. Finally, synthetic cannabinoids (SCs) are human-made (chemically engineered) mind altering chemical agonists that structurally may or may not be similar to naturally occurring phytocannabinoids but are full agonists at cannabinoid receptors, unlike THC which is a partial agonist of CB1 and CB2 receptors [9]. It is the CB1 receptor and its interaction with THC or similar ligands such as SCs that leads to the psychotropic effects. Through antagonistic effects on the CB1 receptor, marijuana induces its mental and behavioral effects. The initial research into biologically active analogs (essentially SCs) were performed by pharmaceutical companies pursuing biological activity but lacking psychoactive side effects. At present, there are two SCs derived from cannabis that are used medically and regulated and those are dronabinol and nabilone [10]. Dronabinol is a scheduled III drug and Nabilone is a schedule II drug with the former used for nausea and vomiting related to chemotherapy, anorexia or AIDS, and the latter is also used for nausea or vomiting from chemotherapy. Unfortunately, underground laboratories have utilized this research and produced illicit compounds used as alternatives for marijuana. The physiology of the human endocannabinoid system makes it possible to be exploited and makes it receptive to exogenous synthetic compounds, making it an easy target for abuse [11].

2. Endocannabinoid system

The endocannabinoid system consists of the endocannabinoids and the cannabinoid receptors. Cannabinoid receptors (CB1) are expressed in the brain, peripheral nervous system and peripheral tissues such as the heart, gut, liver, reproductive system, immune system and the respiratory system [12]. CB2 subtype is expressed in peripheral organs with immune function such as spleen, thymus, tonsils, and in cells such as macrophages and leukocytes. Despite what is known about cannabinoid receptors, what is still subject to debate is the physiologic function of these receptors. Of importance however, is that CB1 receptors are the most prevalent G-protein coupled receptors in the human brain and is highly expressed in cognitive processing regions and in the reward regions of the brain [13]. CB1 and CB2 receptors play a key part in a yet to be fully understood endogenous cannabinoid signaling system. The principal lipid ligands known as anandamide (AEA) and 2-arachidonyl glycerol (2-AG) are responsible for signal transduction but may also themselves be acted upon by specific and important enzymes during signal transduction. Although the components of the endocannabinoid system may remain consistent through life, its function is drastically different during nervous system development as eCB play important roles in neurodevelopment and synaptic plasticity [14, 15]. Unfortunately, it is also under appreciated that brain development does not stop until late adolescence (18–24 years old) [16].

In the brain, the endocannabinoid system is involved in sleep regulation, anxiety control, reward reaction, appetite control, neuroprotection and neural development. During adolescence, eCB and their respective receptors play a vital role in neurodevelopment processes such as pruning and synaptic plasticity [17, 18]. During fetal growth and development and during continued maturation post birth, eCB play an important role in central nervous system (CNS) development with neuro progenitor cells which are multipotent stem cells that can form new cells in the nervous system. So eCB system plays a critical regulatory role throughout development, from the determination of cell fate determined by progenitor cells and neuronal migration to regulation of synaptic transmission and signaling pathways of the fully developed CNS [19]. The precise mechanism by which eCB system molds adolescent brain development however is not clear.

2.1 Psychiatric implications of exogenous THC on the endocannabinoid system

What is clear, however, is that cannabis use is commonly initiated during adolescence and that the exogenous THC psychotropic impact is experienced through the developing eCB system during a vulnerable period of neurodevelopment. One of the concerns, during this neurodevelopment transition period is that marijuana will "over activate" the eCB system resulting in behavioral abnormalities and possibly addiction [7, 20]. Adolescence is a critical time period for brain development which involves the eCB system and there is some evidence noted below that would indicate that this age group's mental health may be particularly vulnerable to the effects of exogenous THC. Some of the behavioral abnormalities that have been linked to cannabis use in younger people, before the age of 17, are schizophrenia, psychosis, bipolar disorders and addiction [15]. More specifically, Goggi and coworkers found that there was an association of cannabis use during adolescence (age $<$ 18 years) and depression, suicidal ideation and suicide attempts [21]. The authors' meta-analysis suggest that cannabis could be a significant factor, among many, contributing to depression in young adulthood and is consistent with the negative influence of cannabis in brain plasticity during development.

Adolescent impulsivity associated with prolonged myelination process and the lack of prefrontal inhibitory control during this period of growth and development could set this population up for some mental health issues precipitated by cannabis. Kristen Schmidt and colleagues [22], in their systematic review of adolescent cannabis use and suicide, found there to be a significant relationship among suicidal thoughts, behavior and suicide attempts with adolescent cannabis users. The UCLA psychiatric group suggests that cannabis is an independent predictor of suicide in this age group and that frequency of cannabis use is associated with increased suicide attempts. Consistent with this finding in adolescents was the study by Hosseini and Oremus from Canada showing earlier age-of-initiation of cannabis use was associated with a higher risk of psychosis [23]. Indeed, early-onset cannabis use (age < 18) but not late onset cannabis use was associated with a higher risk for major depressive disorder by Schoeler and colleagues out of London, especially for individuals with higher frequency cannabis use [24]. Although the causality of cannabis use and mental health issues remain unclear among adolescent studies [25], there are other issues that are also important for clinicians to counsel adolescents and parents regarding cannabis use: cannabis may have detrimental effects on cognition, brain and educational outcomes that can persist beyond acute intoxication and second, improvement of these detrimental effects appear possible with sustained abstinence [26].

2.2 Cannabis use disorder and cannabis withdrawal syndrome

The most frequent negative effect of chronic cannabis exposure is addiction and regular cannabis users may develop a cannabis use disorder called CUD. CUD is defined as the inability to stop consuming cannabis even when it is causing physical or psychological harm, generally including compulsive use and neglect of obligations [27]. In many regular cannabis users, cannabis withdrawal syndrome (CWS) may occur with cessation of cannabis use and is an indicator of CUD. Signs and symptoms of CWS include cravings, irritability, sleep disruption, aggression, weight loss, depression, anxiety, sweating, headaches, tremors and fatigue and may occur within days of stopping cannabis [15]. There are no approved medications for either CUD or CWS. However, initial treatment would be similar to many other withdrawal syndromes. Supportive care and treatment for CWS for those with no prior psychiatric history, has included a tapering dose of phenobarbital (seizures), Escitalopram and low dose benzodiazepines (anxiety), clonidine, (generalized withdrawal symptoms), Naltrexone (cravings), and Metoclopramide (nausea) [28].

Although the temperament of the above information may imply some form of consensus that regular cannabis use during adolescence has uniformly negative consequences for cognitive impairment, the evidence is very complex and evolving and will likely take years to elucidate. For adolescents or young adults who come in for cannabis related toxicity and appear to be "regular or heavy users", the clinician may want to offer advice regarding the potential for adverse cognitive, neural, and educational effects from daily cannabis use [26]. There is some evidence, however, for cognitive recovery after 4–6 weeks of abstinence from cannabis use [29], although there may be some folly in that recommendation to quit as many adolescences and adults who are regular users find it difficult to end their cannabis addiction because of possible neuroadaptation that may occur with regular use [30, 31]. Current evidence would suggest that initiation of cannabis use should be delayed until much later in adolescence, use should be occasional and not daily, high potency marijuana should be low, and use occurs in ways other than smoking [32].

3. Cannabis consumption

THC is the primary psychoactive chemical in cannabis that is responsible for producing the subjective "high", feelings of euphoria, as well as the adverse effects caused by overdosing such as panic, anxiety, paranoia, and psychosis [33, 34]. The somatic or physiologic effects such as changes in heart rate (HR) and Blood pressure (BP) along with increased cardiac output, cardiac workload, and consequently oxygen workload are also an effect of THC [35]. CBD (acid metabolite THC-COOH) is non psychotropic.

In 12th graders, cannabis has the lowest rate of abeyance of all substances used by this age group [36]. In 2018, over 1/3 of 12 graders used cannabis with 28% of 10 graders and 11% of 8th graders also admitting to cannabis use to some extent, with prevalence starting to move downward in 2021 [37]. Now the effects of cannabis legalization on availability and diminished perceived risk, especially by 12th graders, may be associated with increased adolescent cannabis use. Complicating the increased use is the enhanced potency of the cannabis flower of today because of specialized cultivation techniques resulting in at least a threefold increase in THC from 4% in 1995 to 12% in 2014 [38] with some cannabis flower strains containing upwards to 30% [39]. The effect of legalization of Cannabis has reduced prices and increased sales of high potency cannabis products such as edibles, oils, extracts, and waxes containing even higher amounts of THC (> 70%) [40]. Although changes are likely coming regarding marijuana, cannabis is classified as a Schedule 1 drug by the United States Drug Enforcement Agency (USDEA) and therefore is not regulated except for dronabinol, nabilone and CBD.

One of the underappreciated effects of decriminalization and legalization of cannabis is the impact it has on both the unintentional and intentional exposure to infants and young children [41, 42]. Widespread use of cannabis simply translates to greater access to children. In contradistinction to numerous neurologic manifestations of cannabis intoxication in adolescents and young adults, such as mood and attention alterations, acute psychosis, ataxia, tremor, nystagmus, excessive motor activity or muscle relaxation, infants and young children may exhibit primarily impaired consciousness or sudden, unexplained acute encephalopathy. If intoxicants such as cannabis are not considered in the differential along with infectious, trauma, and metabolic dysfunction or dysregulation (hypoglycemia) then this necessitates larger and more invasive workups or procedures that otherwise might be obviated if only a urine tox screen was considered. Many times parents may not be forthcoming in providing information because of social or legal concerns for child abuse and many adults consider cannabis to be harmless [43]. A very recent publication comparing pre versus peri-post legalization of cannabis found children presenting to the emergency department peri-post legalization were significantly more likely to have altered mental status and respiratory involvement that required pediatric intensive care admissions. Additional clinical findings include behavioral changes of the child, ataxia, respiratory depression, seizures, apnea and coma [42].

Regarding psychiatric issues and cannabis, research has shown a dose-dependent linking between THC and psychosis although cause and effect has not been established [44]. Acute cannabis use or intravascular THC administered to normal healthy adults produces psychotomimetic effects similar to that seen in chronic psychosis [45]. In adolescents, cannabis use at 15 years of age is associated with greater likelihood of psychosis later in life but remains unclear if early onset cannabis use is an independent predictor of adverse events later in life. Indeed, most adverse events observed in individuals reporting early-onset use involve frequent and or high potency cannabis use as the most relevant factor [32].

There are many different modes of consumption of cannabis and each comes with its own risks and benefits. It behooves the user to understand, and novice users in particular, need to appreciate the differences that route of exposure can have in the initiation of effects, the duration of psychoactive effects or the intensity of the "high" [46, 47].

4. Smoking and vaping (aerosolization)

The main reason most people smoke cannabis is to experience the so-called high, which typically includes relaxation, some euphoria, perceptual alterations including time distortions and enhancing every day experiences such as eating, watching movies, listening to music and engaging in sex [48]. In a social context, the high could be accompanied by infectious laughter, talkativeness which enhances sociability coinciding with the peak effects within 30 minutes and ending in 1–2 hours [49]. Acute adverse effects of cannabis use include anxiety and panic attacks, psychotic symptoms and automobile accidents due to the effects on coordination, alertness, and judgment [49].

Smoking marijuana leaves or cannabis plant material is, by far, the most popular means by which to obtain the desired psychoactive effects. In Colorado, USA, approximately 2 ounces of marijuana is sufficient to make 50 marijuana cigarettes [50]. Compared to other forms of consumption, such as vaporization, ingestion, transcutaneous, rectal or vaginal routes, smoking generates the most efficient, consistent and instantaneous "high" in delivering THC in a dose dependent manner to the brain. Bioavailability by smoking ranges between 10 and 35% depending upon the regularity of smoking, depth of inhalation, breath hold and puff duration [35]. Combustion (Smoking) which occurs at a higher temperature than aerosolization and can consistently produce a similar level of cannabinoids, is generally the preferred method of delivery for many adolescents [51].

Alternative (non-combusted) methods of aerosolization such as vaporization may be more appealing for some adolescents because of their availability in youth-friendly palatable preparations. The perception of some adolescents is that vaping is more appealing because it is more discreet, healthier, better tasting, less harsh, lower cost, and resulted in better effects [52]. Devices that generate vapor for inhalation of marijuana such as table top and pocket pen devises do so by heating (electronic or otherwise) cannabis products to a vapor that can be inhaled. Even devices such as e-cigarettes that were designed for nicotine can be modified to deliver marijuana products [53]. E-liquids with flavoring can be used to mask the odor of cannabis and make it less detectable [54]. Many of cannabis extracts (oils, vape cartridges, hash) that are vaporized can contain 60% THC, with solid extracts such as wax, budder, shatter, or crumble can exceed 90% [55, 56]. Any of these extracts can be vaporized through an electronic delivery system and e-cigarettes. "Dabbing" which typically involves heating a small amount of extract (dried, concentrated cannabis) either with a tabletop vaporizer (200°C) without combustion (combustion or pyrolysis can destroy a major fraction of THC) by heating a glass rod or nail head with a blowtorch resulting in a vapor to inhale [57]. This can be a complicated method of vaporizing cannabis concentrates that can include a dab rig (modified water pipe for oils and concentrates) a nail attached to the rig to heat the concentrate, a dabber to apply the dab of concentrate to the nail, a dome placed over the nail to contain the vapor, and a blow torch to heat the nail [36]. But dabbing can be simplified with the use of a modified vape pen also known as dab or wax pen. A "dab" is a colloquial name for butane hash oil (BHO) which is a concentrated THC extract generated using butane as a solvent. The concentrate is then vaporized quickly and the user inhales the vapors and swiftly feels the effects. It's unclear if this method of "dabbing" is inherently more dangerous than ingesting or inhaling flower cannabis (smoking) because of the more concentrated extract. These concentrated extracts can be 20–25% THC to upwards of 80% THC in comparison to smoking dried marijuana leaves which is likely 10–20%. Individuals may "dab" anywhere from a few times to 25–50 times in a brief period until the desired effect is obtained [58]. Similar to the adverse effects of smoking marijuana, risks include blackouts, tachycardia, paranoia, and hallucinations.

Hash, is the oldest form of cannabis extract, is composed of purified trichomes (the tiny hair-like outgrowths on cannabis leaves/flower that appear like sugar dusting on the plant) [39]. Inhalable or vaporized plant, oil or extract that is aerosolized by an electronic heating device may be able to generate a higher blood concentration of THC and likely a corresponding subjective effect although vaping devices can vary in their efficiency in delivering the product. It is important to note that the "strength" of a cannabis product often has few, if any, visual cues so the self-made THC/cannabis products obtained on the streets will likely have variable cannabinoid composition [59].

The pharmacokinetics of smoked and vaporized cannabis/THC produce peak blood concentrations within 3–10 minutes after onset of inhaling with THC being detectable in plasma within seconds after the first puff [35]. Both vaporized and smoked THC produce rapid peak blood concentrations in 30–90 minutes that return to baseline within 2–4 hours [39]. The pharmacodynamic onset of inhaled THC is dose related and the self-reported experiences of intoxication match, to some extent, the onset of peak blood concentration. However, because its high lipophilicity, THC is rapidly redistributed to the tissues, including the brain where it produces its neurocognitive effects. The high lipophilicity of THC also contributes to prolong detection in urine for chronic, everyday users. In certain situations, it may be imperative to obtain blood levels of THC as well as to obtain confirmation for detection of marijuana. It's important to know that false positive urine screens for THC are possible and include: medications such as Naproxen, Ibuprofen, Promethazine, Riboflavin, Pantoprazole and Ketoprofen; and some baby shampoos and soaps [20].

4.1 Passive inhalation of cannabis smoke

There is evidence that passive inhalation by an infant can indeed result in toxicity as shown in a 13-month-old who appeared altered and ill [60]. The infant was sleeping in the parent's room where 20 cannabis smokers were engaged in a party for many hours. The infant was subsequently discharged from the hospital and showed marked improvement after 48 hours with just supportive care. Compared to adults, infants have increased minute ventilation relative to their size, which can result in increased absorption. This likely was an enclosed area with poor ventilation and if blood levels and a urine tox screen had been performed on the infant, a THC level and a positive urine screen would have been found. The exposure of the infant to second-hand cannabis smoke is consistent with a systematic review involving passive exposure to second-hand smoke involving adults [61]. In this "meta-analysis", adults passively exposed to increasing amounts of THC from smoked cannabis, will in kind, also report stronger drug effects and higher levels of THC and metabolites can be found in their urine.

5. Cannabis ingestion

Ingestion of "edibles" are food items made with marijuana or oils infused with THC and come in a variety of forms such as baked goods (brownies, muffins and cookies); candies including gummies, caramels, hard candies, and chocolates; lozenges; or infused beverages [62]. Edibles are becoming more popular because the products are more discreet and convenient, produce no smoke or smell, it eliminates the respiratory risk of inhalation (bronchial irritants and carcinogens), generates no secondhand smoke concerns, and it produces a more prolonged and intense psychoactive effect [47]. Many adolescents are less likely to use edibles because they report more negative effects from edibles [51]. Regardless, data appears to indicate that approximately two thirds of adolescents who use cannabis (smoking) also have used edibles [52]. In addition, edibles pose a more unique problem, especially to the unsuspecting or naive, because there are no other foods, appetizing forms or palatable products in which a drug is purposely infused into it generating the final product. Contributing to the possibility of toxicity is the delayed effects when cannabis products are ingested compared to inhalation. Other concerns include accidental ingestions (especially children), and dose titration as edibles can vary in THC within and across products making it difficult among users to estimate the THC concentration that may lead to overconsumption.

The pharmacokinetics of edible cannabis differ from the profile of inhaled cannabis resulting in peak psychoactive effects being delayed hours after ingestion. As noted above, the effects of inhaled cannabis can be felt within 10 minutes, peak blood concentrations within an hour and complete clearance from the blood within 4 hours. Since adolescents or any adult can feel the effects (pharmacodynamics) of inhaled cannabis within minutes, significant toxicity can occur from consuming edibles if the user expects the same time line. When taken orally, THC (Delta-9 THC) undergoes "first pass effect" as the digestive system absorbs and further bio transforms (metabolize) the drug in the liver and in the process, decreases the availability of the active drug (THC) and generates another active equipotent metabolite (11-OH-THC) as well as the inactive carboxylic acid (THC-COOH) [35]. The hydroxylation of THC by the liver cytochrome P450 system to form 11-OH-THC is a potent psychoactive metabolite that readily crosses the blood brain barrier [63], and may be responsible for the stronger and longer lasting drug effects of edibles in comparison to comparable doses of smoked cannabis [64, 65].

The bioavailability of THC when ingested is 10–20% as much of the cannabinoids contained in cannabis are degraded [20]. The process of absorption, metabolism, and re-distribution generates variable time delay in the onset of effects which may result in the adolescent consuming more than initially intended. Although edibles can produce the same dose-related increments in peak THC blood concentrations and subjective high as inhalation, oral THC may take at least 30 minutes to reach significant blood levels with a peak at 3 hours and clearance from the blood at 12 or more hours [35, 39]. Consequently, oral consumers of edibles generally report longer lasting effects of the cannabis than inhalation as well as more intense and unpleasant side effects which can result in significant toxicity [62, 66, 67].

5.1 Cannabis toxicity from ingestion

Cannabis toxicity from edibles probably results in the majority of visits to the health care system simply because it encompasses all age groups, both young and old. The very young, because toddlers are human vacuum cleaners destined to clean up after adults who left their gummy bears within reach, an unsmoked joint or THC resin on the coffee table or half-eaten cannabis cookie on the floor. If 10 to 30 mg of oral THC is the recommended dose for intoxication in an adolescent/young adult, then a cookie containing approximately 100 mgs of THC that a toddler eats could die from respiratory failure [68]. The adolescent or adult comes to the emergency department because of failure to appreciate the differing THC pharmacokinetic profiles of ingestion vs. inhalation and the user consumed the entire edible cookie after not experiencing the initial effects from ¼ of the intended dose of cookie he was to consume but did not because of delayed effects. Now the anxious adolescent who consumed the entire edible cookie is delirious or severely impaired and is experiencing an unexpected adverse effect in need of at least supportive medical care.

The majority of patients seen for cannabis ingestion will not require any treatment [42, 68, 69]. However, compared to toxicity from inhalation (cannabis), cannabis ingestion will be the mode of exposure that most likely will cause concerning signs and symptoms. Adolescents as well as adults were more likely to intentionally ingest edibles due to overconsumption and poor understanding of the delayed effects and experience tachycardia and CNS excitation that ranged from anxiety, paranoia and panic attacks to altered mental status, psychosis, and seizures with benzodiazepines being the most commonly used medication during care [67, 69]. Treatment for cannabis psychosis in the acute stage including agitation, auditory and visual hallucinations included intramuscular antipsychotics (haloperidol and droperidol), oral risperidone and olanzapine, seclusion as well as benzodiazepines [70]. Most of the other minor interventions will be for nausea and vomiting, fluid hydration and supplemental oxygen. There is no antidote for cannabis toxicity and no way to alter or hasten its metabolism, nor to increase its rate of excretion. The majority of these patients were discharged home from the emergency department with some (<10%) needing hospitalization. Clinical findings in older children and adolescents may include psychosis, ataxia, tremors, nystagmus, mood and attention alterations, excessive motor activity and muscle relaxation [43]. Children (<12 years) were more likely to unintentionally ingest edibles at home and experience CNS sedation with a higher risk of ICU admission and an occasional intubation for CNS depression [42, 69]. For children under the age of 6 years, the most common clinical effects from ingestion included, drowsiness or lethargy, ataxia, agitation or irritability and confusion. The less common but serious effects included respiratory depression, coma and seizure [71]. It is important to realize that cannabis intoxication may be life threatening, especially in the very young [72, 73].

Cannabis intoxication in children should be suspected in an afebrile child, previously known to be healthy, with a clinical presentation that includes drowsiness, lethargy, or coma with no focal neurological findings [72]. Most of the other minor interventions will be for nausea and vomiting, fluid hydration and supplemental oxygen. Although edibles being the most commonly ingested substance, other ingested substances included botanical, concentrates and resins.

There are several studies now that are associating the high percentage of THC with a considerable increase in acute toxicity, especially with an increased risk of psychosis [32, 74, 75].

6. Cannabis during pregnancy and breastfeeding

Cannabis-derived drugs (marijuana) are the most widely used illicit drug in pregnancy and is frequently used to minimize the symptoms of morning sickness [76]. Although marijuana is not listed as a known teratogen, it's conceivable that THC, acting through the eCB system could result in perturbations of the developing fetus that could adversely affect neurodevelopment. Cannabis exposure during pregnancy does not cause congenital defects such as mental retardation and developmental disabilities as with fetal alcohol syndrome [77]. Very early in the peri-conception period there is some evidence that in utero cannabis exposure may increase the risk of anencephaly [78], although evidence on possible adverse impacts on fetal development and neonatal outcomes is inconsistent. However, there are studies that implicate cannabis in causing neurological impairment, hyperactivity, poor cognitive function, and changes in dopaminergic receptors in children when exposed in utero [79].

Marijuana constituents do pass freely across the placenta and has been shown to concentrate in breastmilk at levels 8 times of that of plasma THC [80]. Endocannabinoids (AEA and 2-AG) are also found in breast milk [81]. While there is clear data showing cannabinoids are expressed in breast milk, there is no concrete evidence that infants exposed to such breast milk have any potential health effects [82]. Although the pharmacokinetics are known regarding the metabolism and plasma concentration after inhalation, intravenous and oral cannabis administration, less is known about the distribution of cannabinoids in breast milk. There is also a tendency for breast feeding moms to increase their cannabis use during the postpartum period and this increase translates to enhanced levels of THC in breast milk [83]. Because there is so little information on cannabis use during pregnancy and postpartum use while breast feeding, the clinician may want to consider harm reduction approach to reduce cannabis use during pregnancy and postpartum [18]. The perception during pregnancy and with postpartum mothers using cannabis that little harm is to come from cannabis use is simply not known and further research is urgently needed. Lower birthweight of the newborn is associated with smoking marijuana during pregnancy, as is smoking cigarettes [84]. Whether or not the oxidative stress caused by smoke is a mechanism of low birth weight or if it is a direct effect of cigarette or marijuana is not known [85].

7. Synthetic cannabinoids and their related toxicities

Synthetic cannabinoids (SCs) are chemically engineered agonists to the CB1 receptor in the endocannabinoid system and are biochemically similar to THC in its post receptor activity but may be chemically/structurally quite different to the THC molecule making it undetectable in urine drug screens. It emerged in the 1970s when researchers were hopeful in developing new treatments for cancer and were synthesized in academic centers and pharmaceutical industries [4]. It wasn't until

2008 however that investigators first detected the synthetic cannabinoid (JWH-018) in a herbal product that was related to a forensic investigation [5]. Since then, and actually greatly underappreciated before that, SCs have mushroomed in their prevalence and are now readily available on the streets for abuse purposes. SCs are commonly known as synthetic marijuana or synthetic cannabinoid receptor agonists and are sold in brightly colored foil packages and contain finely cut plant material that has been adulterated or 'sprayed" or soaked with SCs. As such, these SCs are not regulated, there are no "good laboratory practice" associated with the production of SCs by clandestine laboratories, and are classified as Schedule I in the United States based on their chemical structures by the USDEA. The dried plant material used for smoking has no inherent psychotropic effects and are solely a vehicle for delivering the synthetic cannabinoid effect. Initially it was the illegality of marijuana that likely motivated the production of SCs by drug distributers and entrepreneurs to produce compounds that could be marketed to users of marijuana or prospective new users to provide a "legal" alternative to marijuana but still with the desired effects including mood elevation, relaxation, euphoria, or creative thinking [86]. It remains to be seen what impact legalization of marijuana may have in the future regarding the continued use of SCs as the toxicities associated with SCs use by younger audiences are greatly underappreciated.

There are likely over 500 SCs that have been introduced into the recreational markets and they are among the most abused psychoactive substances in Europe and United States [79]. The prevalence of synthetic cannabinoid agonists use by adolescents is reported to be less than 2% in 2021, down from 3 to 10% the year before [37]. Most SCs are very potent and are high-efficiency/full agonists of the CB1 receptors unlike THC, which is considered a partial agonist at the CB1 receptor [3]. However, it is important to realize that the similarities in effects between marijuana and SCs are assumed based only on their receptor binding to CB1 and CB2 as no comparison dosing studies have ever been done. Consequently, the toxicities of SCs are likely underappreciated especially when the adverse effects of marijuana are considered low risk beyond the intoxication effects of low potency cannabis [87]. One author estimates that the risk of an emergency room visit is approximately 30-fold higher with SCs than with cannabis [88]. There is evidence that being a partial or a full agonist of the CB1 receptor along with their binding affinities may correlate with the level of exaggerated psychoactivity [89]. Both SCs and THC activate CB1 receptors which trigger the psychotomimetic effects. Speculation is that the adverse effects and unpredictability of SCs stem from the greater affinity for and increased efficacy at the CB1 receptors, compared to THC, but the relationship is complex [44]. Indeed, the full agonist activity and higher potency of the SCs at the SC1 and SC2 receptors may account in part, for their greater toxicities [90] as it has been estimated that SCs may be 5–80 times more potent at the CB1 receptor than natural cannabis [91]. Besides difference in receptor affinities and whether it is a full or partial agonist at the CB1 receptor, there are likely other differences that may assist in explaining greater toxicity with SCs. First, a remarkable difference in metabolism is that THC has only one active metabolite (11-OH-THC) while SCs can have many metabolites that retain binding affinity and activity at the CB1 receptor [92]. Most of the phytocannabinoids such as THC or cannabinol are metabolized through the liver P450s (CYP2C9, CYP2C19, and CYP3A4) while metabolism of SCs is likely through several metabolic pathways including P450s that may generate metabolites that are injurious to tissues. Although both cannabis and SCs go through the cytochrome P450 system that mediate the phase I reaction, much of the similarities in phase II reaction likely end there as most of cannabis undergoes glucuronidation while SCs undergo multiple processes in both phase I and phase II. However, much of the metabolism of SCs have limited data available. Second, when cannabis is smoked or ingested, all of the additional cannabinoids along with various terpenoids are also inhaled which may provide some complementary or synergistic activity, so called entourage effects [33]. As an example, with increasing potency of cannabis there has been a decrease in CBD levels (increasing THC/CBD ratio) which has been implicated in potentially causing health complications, perhaps because of lessoning of the "entourage effects". In abusing SCs, there are no other cannabinoids or terpenoids ingested (but many other chemicals certainly could be ingested with SCs) that could "off set", blunt, modify the activity at the CB1 receptor or provide some neuroprotective effect or some other non-receptor effect, thereby altering the pharmacodynamic full effects of the SCs.

To be clear, SCs are inherently more dangerous, the production of SCs in clandestine labs do not honor the Good Manufacturing Practice regulations so user beware, and the toxicity of SCs can lead to multiple end organ adverse events, including CNS, which can be classified as either physical or psychological effects. Because there are new SCs flooding the markets to avoid the legal system, the likely presence of multiple SCs being ingested at once is likely. No controlled dosing studies have ever been done in humans with SCs, consequently, the pharmacokinetics and pharmacodynamics of SCs are difficult to report with any assurance. Clinicians should suspect the possibility of SCs in an adolescent or young adult who arrives for evaluation with adverse effects similar to cannabis with a neg urine drug screen, including THC. The clinical effects can be highly variable and this diversity of findings may be attributed to the continued variability in composition and concentration of chemicals within SCs [93]. These findings include cardiovascular events, kidney injuries, gastrointestinal problems, neurological events, pulmonary effects, ocular, or psychiatric conditions [3, 86, 94–99]. At present, the unpredictable effects of SCs and the lack of a clear toxidrome to distinguish SCs from other drugs of abuse makes the differential broad and requires the clinician to first eliminate diverse conditions before settling on the possibility of SCs. In addition, it is also unclear whether the below toxicities are due to the SCs parent molecule, metabolites, or contaminants. See **Table 1** for summary of toxicities: synthetic cannabinoids vs. botanical marijuana (Modified from Ford BM, et al) [98].

7.1 Cardiovascular

Tachycardia and hypertension are the most common clinical effects reported. Associated with tachycardia, there can also be cardiac arrythmias, strokes, chest pain, and myocardial infarctions have also been reported even in adolescents and young adults with no previous cardiac issues. Both bradycardia and hypotension are possible. Other than tachycardia, in comparison to toxicity from marijuana, the other associated cardiovascular toxicities from SCs are not generally reported with marijuana. However, myocardial infarctions have been reported in marijuana smokers and appears to be especially noted during the first hour of exposure.

7.2 Kidney injuries

In the settings of acute toxicity from SCs, there have been numerous reports of acute kidney injuries including elevated serum creatinine, proteinuria, hematuria, acute tubular injury and acute tubular nephritis, hypokalemia, and rhabdomyolysis.

	Human cannabinoid toxicities	
	Synthetic cannabinoids	**Botanical marijuana**
Cardiovascular		
Tachycardia	frequent	uncommon
Arrythmias	possible	rare
Hypertension	possible	rare
Chest pain	possible	rare
Myocardial Infarction/Toxicity	possible	uncommon
Renal		
Acute Kidney Injuries	possible	rare
Gastrointestinal		
Nausea	frequent	rare
Vomiting (hyperemesis)	frequent	rare
Neurological		
Euphoria	frequent	frequent
Appetite Stimulation	frequent	frequent
Nystagmus	possible	possible
Slurred Speech	possible	possible
Lethargy/Ataxia	possible	possible
Confusion	frequent	rare
Seizures	possible	rare
Cerebral Ischemia	possible	rare
Panic Attacks	frequent	rare
Memory Issues	uncommon	frequent
Pulmonary		
Acute Resp Distress Syn	possible	rare
Respiratory Depression	possible	possible
Ocular		
Conjunctival hyperemia	common	frequent
Psychiatric		
Hallucinations (vis/aud)	frequent	rare
Delusions	frequent	rare
Excited Delirium	frequent	rare
Psychosis	possible	uncommon
Agitation	frequent	rare
Anxiety	frequent	rare

Table 1.
Human cannabinoid toxicities: Comparison of synthetic cannabinoid toxicities with botanical marijuana by systems.

Other metabolic disturbances have also been noted in SCs including metabolic/respiratory acidosis and alkalosis. Similar to the cardiovascular toxicities, no renal toxic effects have generally been reported from marijuana.

7.3 Gastrointestinal

Nausea and vomiting are frequently reported with toxicity from SCs and has occurred with cannabis although not as frequently. In fact, it remains unclear why cannabis may suppress emesis in some people and appears to induce it in others. There is a phenomenon of cannabinoid hyperemesis syndrome (CHS) or cyclic vomiting syndrome (CVS), that appears mostly with inhalation of cannabis/SCs but has been observed most frequently with SCs. This is the result of chronic abuse and symptomatic relief can be obtained with hot showers. The most effective means to end CVS is through complete cessation of cannabis use which may take 2 weeks of abstinence. Patients being evaluated for this should be monitored for dehydration and kidney issues as well as Mallory-Weiss tears. Intravenous Haloperidol or Droperidol or application of capsaicin cream to the abdomen appear to be the most effective drugs to control nausea as conventional antiemetics do not appear to offer much relief [100]. Abdominal pain, diarrhea, xerostomia have been reported and resolve. Mouth issues including periodontal bone disease with gingival enlargement have also been seen in chronic use in both CBs and cannabis [101]. Hepatotoxicity has been noted with the use of some SCs [102]. Few GI issues have been reported with cannabis other than related to emesis.

7.4 Neurological

There are a multitude of neurological clinical effects that are possible with toxicity from SCs. Some of the neurological toxicity findings are found in both acute effects of cannabis and SCs and these include, euphoria, appetite stimulation, slurred speech, ataxia/lethargy, and nystagmus. Acute toxicity from SCs is more likely to exhibit the following neurological findings in comparison to cannabis: confusion, anxiety, panic attacks, agitation, irritability, and seizures. Very recently, there was a publication citing evidence that cannabis may have proconvulsant effects [103]. In addition, the following have been reported in acute toxicity from SCs including self-mutilation, catatonia or psychomotor retardation, and memory disturbances. It should be noted that memory disturbances are commonly observed in cannabis abuse.

7.5 Pulmonary

Severe respiratory depression or tachypnea has been observed, along with pneumothorax and acute respiratory distress syndrome can occur with SCs use. In 2019, there was an outbreak of product use-associated lung injury (so called e-cigarette, or vaping, product use associated lung injury, EVALI) [54]. It was not found to be from any particular cannabis or cannabis extact or SCs, but rather from Vitamin E acetate, a diluent and thickening agent in cannabis-based products. Severe respiratory depression can certainly occur with cannabis ingestion as noted above, especially in toddlers and children. Pneumothorax can also occur from both cannabis and SCs use and may be more of a function in maximizing pulmonary absorption by taking very deep and prolonged breaths. Someone with panic attacks or anxiety may be overlooked when an astute clinician or a chest xray may reveal a reason for their anxiety or panic attack and that is a pneumothorax.

7.6 Ocular

Conjunctival hyperemia and mydriasis have been noted in both toxicity from SCs and cannabis.

7.7 Psychiatric

Hallucinations (visual and auditory), anxiety, delusions, excited delirium, and psychosis in susceptible individuals have been noted to be more common in SCs users than in cannabis users regarding acute effects. Psychosis is a condition in which the individual is not able to think clearly, unable to distinguish between reality and false beliefs or delusions. Similar to psychosis with high potency THC, there may be a dose effect that exists for SCs although research is lacking for SCs and absolute confirmation linking cause and effect regarding THC and psychosis is lacking.

As noted above under "neurological", more individuals with toxicity from SCs were found to have confusion, anxiety, agitation, irritability, and panic attacks compared to cannabis users [104]. Suicidal thoughts and attempts have also been noted in toxicity from SCs. In some, the overall effects of SCs can resemble those of cannabis, but those presenting to the hospital are doing so because of behavioral abnormalities (agitation, psychosis or severe anxiety) or because of acute illnesses such as those listed above involving other end organs. Psychosis or psychosis-like conditions appear relatively frequently with the use of SCs and may be a direct or indirect effect (parent SCs or metabolites) of their high potency or perhaps due to the absence of CBD, the so-called entourage effect with marijuana. There is now evidence that SCs exposure in adolescents is associated with higher odds of neuropsychiatric morbidity than cannabis exposure [105].

7.8 Clinical treatment

Clinical management frequently involves supportive care, intravenous fluids, electrolyte replenishment, benzodiazepines for seizures, neuroleptics (Haldol or Droperidol) for psychotic symptoms, or agitation not responsive to benzodiazepines. Many patients may need to be admitted if unstable, or if acute agitation/psychosis is not clearing. In most patients, the effects noted above are not life threatening and generally cease in around 8 hours after consumption [106]. It should also be noted that unlike cannabis, SCs are not detected by common urine drug screens.

8. Conclusion

Cannabis use is long standing and is not going away. There are currently two major driving forces that may dictate the health of a subset of our adolescence if allowed. First, are the socioeconomic and legislative changes that are generating cheaper and legally available cannabis products, perhaps under the guise of a falsely reassuring perception in lack of harm. The second driving force that is also concerning is higher potency cannabinoids, whether they be botanically derived or synthetic in derivation, that acutely cause toxicity in the CNS and other end organs where cannabinoid receptors are abundantly expressed and has been discussed in this review with management recommendations. With continued use, cannabinoid agonists may be linked to poor social and behavioral outcomes later in life as well as neurocognitive deficits yet to be determined. The research is lacking, urgently needed, and findings likely subtle and difficult to quantify. The nature of adolescence and young adulthood is experimentation and risk taking but the involvement of the eCB system may now be unlocked during critical periods of neurodevelopment. Exogenous cannabinoid agonists may lead to exaggerated psychoactive effects that could result in the formation of permanent and irreversible neural networks posing issues later in life. Future vulnerabilities may include cannabis use disorder and withdrawal issues in the short term and psychosis, schizophrenia, and addiction in the long term.

Acknowledgements

Much appreciation to Renee Lamoureux and the librarian staff at Essentiahealth, St. Mary's Hospital, Duluth, Minnesota, USA for their tremendous assistance in completing this manuscript.

Author details

Peter B. Chase
Essentiahealth, Duluth, Minnesota, USA

*Address all correspondence to: pbchasetox@gmail.com

References

[1] Turgeman I, Bar-Sela G. Cannabis use in palliative oncology: A review of the evidence for popular indications. The Israel Medical Association Journal. 2017;**19**:85-88

[2] Mechoulam R. Plant cannabinoids: A neglected pharmacological treasure trove. British Journal of Pharmacology. 2005;**146**:913-915. DOI: 10.1038/sj.bjp.0706415

[3] Alves V, Goncalves J, Aguiar J. The synthetic cannabinoids phenomenon: From structure to toxicological properties. A review. Critical Reviews in Toxicology. 2020;**50**(5):359-382. DOI: 10.1080/10408444.2020.1762539

[4] Papaseit E, Perez-Mana C, Perez-Acevedo A. Cannabinoids: From pot to lab. International Journal of Medical Sciences. 2018;**15**:1286-1295. DOI: 10.7150/ijms.27087

[5] Lafaye G, Karila L, Belcha L. Cannabis, cannabinoid and health. Dialogues in Clinical Neuroscience. 2017;**19**:309-316. DOI: 10.31887/DCNS.2017.19.3/glafaye

[6] Chandra S, Radwan M, Majumdar C, et al. New trends in cannabis potency in USA and Europe during the last decade (2008-2017). European Archives of Psychiatry and Clinical Neuroscience. 2019;**269**:5-15. DOI: 10.1007/s00406-019-00983-5

[7] Iversen L. Cannabis and the brain. Brain. 2003;**126**:1252-1270. DOI: 10.1093/brain/awg143

[8] Mato S, DelOlmo E, Pazos A. Ontogenetic development of cannabinoid receptor expression and signal transduction functionality in the human brain. The European Journal of Neuroscience. 2003;**17**:1747-1754. DOI: 10.1046/j.1460-9568.2003.02599.x

[9] Pertwee R. The diverse CB1 and CB2 receptor pharmacology of three plant cannabinoids: Delta-9 tetrahydrocannabinol, cannabidiol, and delta-9 tetrahydrocannabivarin. British Journal of Pharmacology. 2008;**153**:199-215. DOI: 10.1038/sj.bjp.0707442

[10] Dharmapuri S, Miller K, Klein JD. Marijuana and the pediatric population. Pediatrics. 2020;**146**:e20192629. DOI: 10.1542/peds.2019-2629

[11] Zou S, Kumar U. Cannabinoid receptors and the endocannabinoid system: Signaling and function in the central nervous system. International Journal of Molecular Sciences. 2018;**19**:833. DOI: 10.3390/ijms19030833

[12] Dhein S. Different effects of cannabis abuse on adolescent and adult brain. Pharmacology. 2020;**105**:609-617. DOI: 10.1159/000509377

[13] Mechoulam R, Parker L. The endocannabinoid system and the brain. Annual Review of Psychology. 2013;**64**:21-47. DOI: 10.1146/annurev-psych-113011-143739

[14] Farrelly AM, Vlachou S. Effects of cannabinoid exposure during neurodevelopment on future effects of drugs of abuse: A preclinical perspective. International Journal of Molecular Sciences. 2021;**22**(18):9989. DOI: 10.3390/ijms22189989

[15] Augustin SM, Lovinger DM. Synaptic changes induced by cannabinoid drugs and cannabis use disorder. Neurobiology

of Disease. 2022;**167**:105670. DOI: 10.1016/j.nbd.2022.105670

[16] Johnson S, Blum R, Giedd J. Adolescent maturity and the brain: The promise and pitfalls of neuroscience research in adolescent health policy. The Journal of Adolescent Health. 2009;**45**:216-221. DOI: 10.1016/j.jadohealth.2009.05.016

[17] Meyers H, Francis S, Dylan G. The role of the endocannabinoid system and genetic variation in adolescent brain development. Neuropsychopharmacology. 2018;**43**:21-33. DOI: 10.1038/npp.2017.143

[18] O'Dell CP, Tuell DS, Shah DS, Stone WL. The systems medicine of cannabinoids in pediatrics: The case for more pediatric studies. Frontiers in Bioscience (Landmark Ed). 2022;**27**:14. DOI: 10.31083/j.fbl2701014

[19] Bara A, Ferland J, Rompala G. Cannabis and synaptic reprograming of the developing brain. Nature Reviews. Neuroscience. 2021;**22**:423-438. DOI: 10.1038/s41583-021-00465-5

[20] Miller NS, Oberbarnscheidt T. Pharmacology of marijuana. Journal of Addiction Research & Therapy. 2016;**S11**:012. DOI: 10.4172/2166-6105.1000S11-012

[21] Gobbi G, Atkin T, Zytynski T. Association of cannabis use in adolescence risk of depression, anxiety, and suicidality in young adults. JAMA Psychiatry. 2019;**76**(4):426-434

[22] Schimdt K, Tseng I, Phan A. A systematic review: Adolescent cannabis use and suicide. Addictive Disorders and Their Treatment. 2020;**19**(3):146-151. DOI: 10.1097/ADT.0000000000000196

[23] Hosseini S, Oremus M. The effect of age of initiation of cannabis use on psychosis, depression, anxiety among youth under 25 years. The Canadian Journal of Psychiatry. 2019;**64**(5):304-312. DOI: 10.1177/0706743718809339

[24] Schoeler T, Theobald D, Pingault JP. Developmental sensitivity to cannabis use patterns and risk for major depressive disorder in mid-life: Findings from 40 years of follow-up. Psychological Medicine. 2018;**16**(22):32. DOI: 10.1017/SO033291717003658

[25] Cancilliere MK, Yusufov M, Weyandt L. Effects of co-occurring marijuana use and anxiety on brain structure and functioning: A systematic review of adolescent studies. Journal of Adolescence. 2018;**65**:177-188

[26] Lorenzetti V, Hoch E, Hall W. Adolescent cannabis use, cognition, brain health and educational outcomes: A review of the evidence. European Neuropsychopharmacology. 2020;**36**:169-180

[27] Connor JP, Stjepanovic D, Le Foll B. Cannabis use and cannabis use disorder. Nature Reviews. Disease Primers. 2021;**7**:16. DOI: 10.1038/s41572-021-00247-4

[28] Cooper ZD. Adverse effects of synthetic cannabinoids: Management of acute toxicity and withdrawal. Current Psychiatry Reports. 2016;**18**:52. DOI: 10.1007/s11920-016-0694-1

[29] Scott JC, Slomiak ST, Jones JD. Association of cannabis with cognitive functioning in adolescents and young adults: A systematic review and meta-analysis. JAMA Psychiatry. 2018;**75**:585-595. DOI: 10.1001/jamapsychiatry.2018.0335

[30] Volkow ND, Koob GF, Mclellan AT. Neurobiologic advances from the brain disease model of addiction. The

New England Journal of Medicine. 2016;**374**:363-371. DOI: 10.1056/NEJMra1511480

[31] Zehra A, Burns J, Kure LC. Cannabis addiction and the brain: A review. Journal of Neuroimmune Pharmacology. 2018;**13**:438-452. DOI: 10.1007/s11481-018-9782-9

[32] Fischer B, Robinson T, Bullen C. Lower-risk cannabis use guidelines (LRCUG) for reducing health harms from non-medical cannabis use: A comprehensive evidence and recommendation update. International Journal of Drug Policy. 2022;**99**:103381. DOI: 10.1016/j.drugpo.2021.103381

[33] Russo EB. Taming THC: Potential cannabis synergy and phytocannabinoid-terpenoid entourage effects. British Journal of Pharmacology. 2011;**163**:1344-1364. DOI: 10.1111/j.1476-5381.2011.01238.x

[34] Schlienz NJ, Spindle TR, Cone EJ. Pharmacodynamic dose effects of oral cannabis ingestion in healthy adults who infrequently use cannabis. Drug and Alcohol Dependence. 2020;**211**:107969. DOI: 10.1016/j.drugalcdep.2020.107969

[35] Grotenhermen F. Pharmacokinetics and pharmacodynamics of cannabinoids. Clinical Pharmacokinetics. 2003;**42**:327-360. DOI: 10.2165/00003088-200342040-00003

[36] Struble CA, Ellis JD, Lundahl LH. Beyond the bud: Emerging methods of cannabis consumption for youth. Pediatric Clinics of North America. 2019;**66**:1087-1097. DOI: 10.1016/j.pcl.2019.08.012

[37] Johnston LD, Meich RA, O'Malley PM. Monitoring the Future National Survey Results on Drug Use 1975-2021: Overview, Key Findings on Adolescent Drug Use. Ann Arbor (MI): Institute For Social Research, The University of Michigan; 2022

[38] ElSohly MA, Mehmedic Z, Foster S. Changes in cannabis potency over the last 2 decades (1995-2014): Analysis of current data in the United States. Biological Psychiatry. 2016;**79**:613-619. DOI: 10.1016/j.biopsych.2016.01.004

[39] Ramaekers JG, Mason NL, Kloft L. The why behind the high: Determinants of neurocognition during acute cannabis exposure. Nature Reviews. Neuroscience. 2021;**22**:439-454. DOI: 10.1038/s41583-021-00466-4

[40] Smart R, Caulkins JP, Kilmer B. Variation in cannabis potency and prices in a newly legal market: Evidence from 30 million cannabis sales in Washington state. Addiction. 2017;**112**:2167-2177. DOI: 10.1111/add.13886

[41] Wang GS, LeLait MC, Keakyne SJ. Unintentional pediatric exposures to marijuana in Colorado, 2009-2015. JAMA Pediatrics. 2016;**170**:e160971. DOI: 10.1001/jamapediatrics.2016.0971

[42] Cohen N, Blanco LG, Davis A. Pediatric cannabis intoxication trends in the pre and post-legalization era. Clinical Toxicology. 2022;**60**:53-58. DOI: 10.1080/15563650.2021.1939881

[43] Lavi E, Rekhtman D, Berkun Y. Sudden onset unexplained encephalopathy in infants: Think of cannabis intoxication. European Journal of Pediatrics. 2016;**175**:417-420. DOI: 10.1007/s00431-015-2639-9

[44] Deng H, Verrico CD, Kosten TR. Psychosis and synthetic cannabinoids. Psychiatry Research. 2018;**268**:400-412. DOI: 10.1016/j.psychres.2018.08.012

[45] D'Souza DC, Perry E, MacDougall L. The psychotomimetic effects

of intravenous Dleta-9-tetrahydrocannabinol in healthy individuals: Implications for psychosis. Neuropsychopharmacology. 2004;**29**:1558-1572. DOI: 10.1038/sj.npp.1300496

[46] Borodovsky JT, Crosier BS, Lee DC. Smoking, vaping eating: Is legalization impacting the way people use cannabis? The International Journal on Drug Policy. 2016;**36**:141-147. DOI: 10.1016/j.drugpo.2016.02.022

[47] Doran N, Papadopoulos A. Cannabis edibles: Behaviours, attitudes, and reasons for use. Environmental Health Review. 2019;**62**:44-52. DOI: 10.5864/d2019-011

[48] Green B, Kavanagh D, Young R. Being stoned: A review of self-reported cannabis effects. Drug and Alcohol Review. 2003;**22**:453-460. DOI: 10.1080/09595230310001613976

[49] Hall W, Degenhardt L. Adverse health effects of non-medical cannabis use. Lancet. 2009;**374**:1383-1391. DOI: 10.1016/S0140-6736(09)610370

[50] Ghosh TS, Van Dyke M, Maffey A. Medical Marijuana's public health lessons-implications for retail marijuana in Colorado. The New England Journal of Medicine. 2015;**372**:991-993. DOI: 10.1056/NEJMp1500043

[51] Boisvert EE, Bae D, Pang RD. Subjective effects of combustible, vaporized, and edible cannabis: Result from a survey of adolescent cannabis users. Drug and Acohol Dependence. 2020;**206**:107716. DOI: 10.1016/j.drugalcdep.2019.107716

[52] Knapp AA, Lee DC, Borodovsky JT. Emerging trends in cannabis administration among adolescent cannabis users. The Journal of Adolescent Health. 2019;**64**:487-493. DOI: 10.1016/j.jadohealth.2018.07.012

[53] Stefaniak AB, LeBouf RF, Ranpara AC. Toxicology of flavoring- and cannabis-containing e-liquids used in electronic delivery systems. Pharmacology & Therapeutics. 2021;**224**:107838. DOI: 10.1016/j.pharmthera.2021.107838

[54] Blount BC, Karwowski MP, Shields PG. Vitamin E acetate in bronchoalveolar-lavage fluid associated with EVALI. The New England Journal of Medicine. 2020;**382**:697-705. DOI: 10.1056/NEJMoa1916433

[55] Caulkins JP, Bao Y, Davenport S. Big data on big new market: Insights from Washington State's legal cannabis market. The International Journal on Drug Policy. 2018;**57**:86-94. DOI: 10.1016/j.drugpo.2018.03.031

[56] Cavazos-Rehg PA, Krauss MJ, Sowles SJ. Leveraging user perspectives for insight into cannabis concentrates. The American Journal of Drug and Alcohol Abuse. 2018;**44**(6):628-641. DOI: 10.1080/00952990.2018.1436179

[57] Loflin M, Eareleywine M. A new method of cannabis ingestion: The dangers of dabs? Addictive Behaviors. 2014;**39**:1430-1433. DOI: 10.1016/j.addbeh.2014.05.013

[58] Krauss MJ, Sowles SJ, Mylvaganam S. Displays of dabbing marijuana extracts on YouTube. Drug and Alcohol Dependence. 2015;**155**:45-51. DOI: 10.1016/j.drugalcdep.2015.08.020

[59] Hammand D. Communicating THC levels and 'dose' to consumers: Information for product labelling and packaging of cannabis products in regulated markets. The International Journal on Drug Policy.

2021;**91**:102509. DOI: DOI.org/10.1016/j.drugpo.2019.07.004

[60] Zarfin Y, Yefet E, Abozaid S. Infant with altered consciousness after cannabis passive inhalation. Child Abuse and Neglect. 2012;**36**:81-83. DOI: 10.1016/j.chiabu.2011.09.011

[61] Holitzki H, Dowsett LE, Spackman E. Health effects of exposure to second and third-hand marijuana smoke: A systematic review. CMAJ Open. 2017;**5**:E814-E822. DOI: 10.9778/cmajo.20170112

[62] Giombi KC, Kosa KM, Rains C. Consumers' perspective of edible marijuana products for recreational use: Likes, dislikes, and reasons for use. Substance Use & Misuse. 2018;**53**(4):541-547. DOI: 10.1080/10826084.2017.1343353

[63] Mura P, Kintz P, Dumestre V. THC can be detected in brain while absent in blood. Journal of Analytical Toxicology. 2005;**29**:842-843. DOI: 10.1093/jat/29.8.842

[64] Favrat B, Menetrey A, Augsburger M. Two cases of "cannabis acute psychosis" following the administration of oral cannabis. BMC Psychiatry. 2005;**5**:17. DOI: 10.1186/1471-244X-5-17

[65] Barrus DG, Capogrossi KL, Cates SC. Tasty THC: Promises and Challenges of Cannabis Edibles. RTI Press; 2016. DOI: 10.3768/rtipress.2016.op.0035.1611

[66] Lamy FR, Daniulaityte R, Sheth A. "Those edibles hit hard": Exploration of twitter data on cannabis edibles in the US. Drug and Alcohol Dependence. 2016;**164**:64-70. DOI: 10.1016/j.drugalcdep.2016.04.029

[67] Monte AA, Shelton SK, Mills E. Acute illness associated with cannabis use, by route of exposure: An observational study. Annals of Internal Medicine. 2019;**170**:531-537. DOI: 10.7326/M18-2809

[68] Monte AA, Zane RD, Heard KJ. The implications of marijuana legalization in Colorado. Journal of the American Medical Association. 2015;**313**:241-242. DOI: 10.1001/jama.2014.17057

[69] Noble MJ, Hedberg K, Hendrickson RG. Acute cannabis toxicity. Clinical Toxicology. 2019;**57**:735-742. DOI: 10.1080/15563650.2018.1548708

[70] Hudak M, Severn D, Nordstrom K. Edible cannabis-induced psychosis: Intoxication and beyond. The American Journal of Psychiatry. 2015;**172**:911-912. DOI: 10.1176/appi.ajp.2015.15030358

[71] Onders B, Casavant MJ, Spiller HA. Marijuana exposure among children younger than six years in the United States. La Clinica Pediatrica. 2016;**55**(5):428-436. DOI: 10.1177/0009922815589912

[72] Claudet I, Le Breton M, Brehin C. A 10-year review of cannabis exposure in children under 3-years of age: Do we need a more global approach? European Journal of Pediatrics. 2017;**176**:553-556. DOI: 10.1007/s00431-017-2872-5

[73] Pelissier F, Claudet I, Pelissier-Alicot AL. Parental cannabis abuse and accidental intoxications in children. Pediatric Emergency Care. 2014;**30**:862-866. DOI: 10.1097/PEC.0000000000000288

[74] Blithikioti C, Miquel L, Batalla A. Cerebellar alterations in cannabis users: A systematic review. Addiction Biology. 2019;**24**:1121-1137. DOI: 10.1111/adb.12714

[75] Kroon E, Kuhns L, Hoch E. Heavy cannabis use, dependence and the

brain: A clinical perspective. Addiction. 2019;**115**:559-572. DOI: 10.1111/add.14776

[76] Agrawal A, Grucza RA, Rogers CE. Public health implications of rising marijuana use in pregnancy in an age of increasing legalization. JAMA Pediatrics. 2019;**173**:607. DOI: 10.1001/jamapediatrics.2019.0618

[77] Hurd YL. Cannabis and the developing brain challenge risk perception. The Journal of Clinical Investigation. 2020;**130**:3947-3949. DOI: 10.1172/JCI139051

[78] van Gelder MM, Donders AR, Devine O. Using Bayesian models to assess the effects of under-reporting of cannabis use on the association with birth defects, national birth defects prevention study, 1997-2005. Paediatric and Perinatal Epidemiology. 2014;**28**:424-433. DOI: 10.1111/ppe.12140

[79] Chung EY, Cha HJ, Min HK. Pharmacology and adverse effects of new psychoactive substances: Synthetic cannabinoid receptor agonists. Archives of Pharmacal Research. 2021;**44**:402-413. DOI: 10.1007/s12272-021-01326-6

[80] Perez-Reyes M, Wall ME. Presence of delta9-tetrahydrocannabinol in human milk. The New England Journal of Medicine. 1982;**307**:819-820. DOI: 10.1056/NEJM198209233071311

[81] Di Marzo V, De Petrocellis L, Mechoulam R. Trick or treat from food endocannabinoids? Nature. 1998;**396**:636-637. DOI: 10.1038/25267

[82] Baker T, Datta P, Rewers-Felkins K, Thompson H. Transfer of inhaled cannabis into human breast Milk. Obstetrics and Gynecology. 2018;**131**:783-788. DOI: 10.1097/AOG.0000000000002575

[83] Moss MJ, Bushlin I, Kazmierczak S. Cannabis use and measurement of cannabinoids in plasma breast milk of breastfeeding mothers. Pediatric Research. 2021;**90**:861-868. DOI: 10.1038/s41390-020-01332-2

[84] Crume TL, Juhl AL, Brooks-Russell A. Cannabis use during the perinatal period in a state with legalized recreational and medical marijuana: The association between maternal characteristics, breastfeeding patterns, and neonatal outcomes. The Journal of Pediatrics. 2018;**197**:90-96. DOI: 10.1016/j.jpeds.2018.02.005

[85] Stone WL, Bailey B, Khraisha N. The pathophysiology of smoking during pregnancy: A systems biology approach. Frontiers in Bioscience. 2014;**6**:318-328. DOI: 10.2741/e708

[86] Gurney SM, Scott KS, Kacinko SL. Pharmacology, toxicology, and adverse effects of synthetic cannabinoid drugs. Forensic Science Review. 2014;**26**:54-78

[87] Sumnall HR, Evans-Brown M, McVeigh J. Social, policy, and public health perspectives on new psychoactive substances. Drug Testing and Analysis. 2011;**3**:515-523. DOI: 10.1002/dta.310

[88] Martinotti G, Santacroce R, Papanti D. Synthetic Cannabinoids: psychopharmacology, clinical aspects, and psychotic onset. CNS & Neurological Disorders Drug Targets. 2017;**16**:567-575. DOI: 10.2174/1871527316666170413101839

[89] Su MK, Seely KA, Moran JH. Metabolism of classical cannabinoids and the synthetic cannabinoid JWH-018. Clinical Pharmacology and Therapeutics. 2015;**97**:562-564. DOI: 10.1002/cpt.114

[90] Pintori N, Loi B, Mereu M. Synthetic cannabinoids: The hidden side of spice drugs. Behavioural Pharmacology.

2017;**28**:409-419. DOI: 10.1097/FBP.0000000000000323

[91] Adams AJ, Banister SD, Irizarry L. "Zombie" outbreak caused by the synthetic cannabinoid AMB-FUBINACA in New York. The New England Journal of Medicine. 2017;**376**:235-242. DOI: 10.1056/NEJMoa1610300

[92] Rajasekaran M, Brents LK, Franks LN. Human metabolites of synthetic cannabinoids JWH-018 and JWH-073 bind with high affinity and act as potent agonists at cannabinoid type-2 receptors. Toxicology and Applied Pharmacology. 2013;**269**:100-108. DOI: 10.1016/j.taap.2013.03.012

[93] Kasper AM, Ridpath AD, Gerona RR. Severe illness associated with reported use of synthetic cannabinoids: A public health investigation (Mississippi, 2015). Clinical Toxicology (Philadelphia, Pa.). 2019;**75**:10-18. DOI: 10.1080/15563650.2018.1485927

[94] Tait RJ, Caldicott D, Mountain D. A systematic review of adverse events arising from the use of synthetic cannabinoids and their associated treatment. Clinical Toxicology (Philadelphia, Pa.). 2016;**54**:1-13. DOI: 10.3109/15563650.2015.1110590

[95] Rajashekare RY, Mekala HM, Sidhu M. Synthetic cannabinoids—"spice" can induce a psychosis: A brief review. Innovations in Clinical Neuroscience. 2019;**16**:31-32

[96] Courts J, Maskill V, Gray A. Signs and symptoms associated with synthetic cannabinoid toxicity: Systematic review. Australasian Psychiatry. 2016;**24**:598-601. DOI: 10.1177/1039856216663733

[97] Bukke VN, Archana M, Villani R. Pharmacological and toxicological effects of phytocannabinoids and recreational synthetic cannabinoids: Increasing risk of public health. Pharmaceuticals (Basel). 2021;**14**:965. DOI: 10.3390/ph14100965

[98] Ford BM, Tai S, Fantegrossi WE. Synthetic pot: Not your Grandfather's marijuana. Trends in Pharmacological Sciences. 2017;**38**:257-276. DOI: 10.1016/j.tips.2016.12.003

[99] Tournebize J, Gibaja V, Kahn JP. Acute effects of synthetic cannabinoids: Update 2015. Substance Abuse. 2017;**38**:344-366. DOI: 10.1080/08897077.2016.1219438

[100] Schep LJ, Slaughter RJ, Glue P. The clinical toxicology of cannabis. The New Zealand Medical Journal. 2020;**133**:96-103

[101] Momen-Heravi F, Kang P. Management of cannabis-induced periodontitis via resective surgical therapy. Journal of the American Dental Association. 2017;**148**:179-184. DOI: 10.1016/j.adaj.2016.10.009

[102] Solimini R, Busardo FP, Rotolo MC. Hepatotoxicity associated to synthetic cannabinoids use. European Review for Medical and Pharmacological Sciences. 2017;**21**:1-6

[103] Kaczor EE, Greene G, Zacharia J. The potential proconvulsant effects of cannabis: A scoping review. Journal of Medical Toxicology. 2022;**18**:223-234. DOI: 10.1007/s13181-022-00886-3

[104] Chase PB, Hawkins J, Mosier J. Differential physiological and behavioral cues observed in individuals smoking botanical marijuana versus synthetic cannabinoid drugs. Clinical Toxicology (Philadelphia, Pa.). 2016;**54**:14-19. DOI: 10.3109/15563650.2015.1101769

[105] Anderson SA, Oprescu AM, Calello DP. Neuropsychiatric sequelae in adolescents with acute synthetic cannabinoid toxicity. Pediatrics. 2019;**144**:e20182690. DOI: 10.1542/peds.2018-2690

[106] Correia B, Fernandes J, Botica MJ. Novel psychoactive substances: The razor's edge between therapeutical potential and psychoactive recreational misuse. Medicine. 2022;**9**:19. DOI: 10.3390/medicines9030019

Chapter 6

Evidence of Health Effects Associated with Marijuana Use: A Comprehensive Public Health Review

Richard Holdman

Abstract

Starting in 2014, Colorado Department of Public Health was designated to monitor the emerging science and medical information relevant to the health effects associated with marijuana use. After years of conducting an ongoing systematic review of scientific literature, we have established 139 evidence statements within 11 health topics. Our mission is to translate the science into meaningful public health statements and recommendations to inform and educate the general public, healthcare providers, and everyone in-between on the health effects associated with marijuana use. This chapter summarizes evidence from all of our health topics; ranging from respiratory effects of marijuana to cognitive and academic effects of marijuana use on adolescents and young adults.

Keywords: tetrahydrocannabinol, marijuana use, health effects, public health, systematic review

1. Introduction

In 2014 recreational, adult-use of cannabis (interchangeably referred to as marijuana) was established in the state of Colorado. At this time the Colorado Department of Public Health and Environment (CDPHE) was given statutory responsibility in Colorado Revised Statute (C.R.S.) 25-1.5-110, to; "monitor changes ... in the emerging science and medical information relevant to the health effects associated with marijuana use." and "appoint a panel of health care professionals with expertise in, but not limited to, neuroscience, epidemiology, toxicology, cannabis physiology, and cannabis quality control to further direct policy." Based on this charge, CDPHE appointed a 14-member committee titled the Retail Marijuana Public Health Advisory Committee (RMPHAC) to review scientific literature on the health effects of marijuana.

Under the same statute mentioned previously, the RMPHAC is directed to "... establish criteria for studies to be reviewed, reviewing studies and other data, and making recommendations, as appropriate, for policies intended to protect consumers of marijuana or marijuana products and the general public." To implement this charge, the RMPHAC meets four or five times a year to review the scientific literature currently available on health effects of marijuana use, evaluate findings without bias, openly discuss the science and apply expert opinion, come to consensus on the science, translate the science into public health messages, make policy-related recommendations, recommend surveillance activities, and identify and address gaps in the science important to public health. All this information is compiled and detailed in a report every two years for the Colorado State Board of Health, the Colorado Department of Revenue, and the Colorado General Assembly, titled "Monitoring Health Concerns Related to Marijuana in Colorado" [1].

Since 2014, and prior to this publication, the RMPHAC has come together on a quarterly basis, held discussions concerning hundreds of articles, and developed over one hundred evidence statements within eleven health topics. As more scientific evidence regarding cannabis health effects are published, this committee continues to build upon existing evidence statements or will construct new statements when appropriate. This chapter will detail the review methods used by the RMPHAC to develop evidence statements about the health effects associated with marijuana use, describe the findings from all eleven health topics, and report the public health statements, recommendations, and research gaps used to inform public health policy in the State of Colorado.

2. Systematic review development and process

The first step in the process of investigating the health effects from marijuana use was to develop and implement an unbiased, transparent, and complete process for evaluating scientific literature and data on marijuana use and health outcomes. To ensure this, the RMPHAC and CDPHE technical staff developed a twelve step review process guided by the established preferred reporting items for systematic reviews and meta-analyses (PRISMA) framework [2]. These twelve steps are followed for each review and are as follows:

1. Conduct a broad search of current peer-reviewed publications quarterly. Relevant articles cited in reviews or other primary studies are also included.

2. Review relevant full-text articles identified in the search.

3. Rate the findings: each finding in the articles is rated as a high-, medium-, or low-quality finding based on strengths and limitations of the methods. Evaluation of the strengths and limitations was based on criteria in the grading of recommendations assessment, development and evaluation (GRADE) system, a well-accepted method for evaluating the quality of scientific evidence [3].

4. Group related findings: each finding is categorized based on population, exposure, and outcome (health effect), to answer specific questions.

5. Weigh the evidence: draft evidence statements that summarize the quantity and quality of evidence answering a specific question.

6. Translate the evidence: draft public health statement that translate the evidence statement into language at an 11th grade reading level.

7. Synthesize the evidence: draft public health recommendations (e.g., for education or monitoring) based on important information identified through the review process.

8. Identify research gaps: draft statements to articulate the research gaps identified during the review process.

9. Present to committee: findings, evidence statements, public health statements, public health recommendations, and research gaps are publicly presented to the RMPHAC for review and revision during open public meetings.

10. Public comment: during the open public meetings, interested stakeholders and members of the public are invited to provide comments relevant to the topics presented.

11. Reach consensus: committee members come to consensus on findings, evidence statement, public health statement, public health recommendations, and research gaps.

12. Adopt summary statements: committee votes to officially accept findings, evidence statements, public health statements, public health recommendations, and research gaps.

All review methods were approved by the RMPHAC, including the terms used to conduct the ongoing broad search of peer-reviewed publications for relevant literature. Medline is the priority research database used to obtain articles for review. Embase, the biomedical database, and gray literature were secondarily reviewed when references in included articles were not included in Medline searches. Studies of marijuana use in humans were the primary focus of the review, with animal studies included for only specific topics with limited human research. All identified peer-reviewed literature on a given topic was reviewed, regardless of positive or negative findings or quality of the methods utilized. For the ongoing broad Medline search, medical subject heading (MeSH) terms were used and is as follows; "Cannabis"[Mesh] OR Marijuana "Smoking"[Mesh] OR "Marijuana Abuse"[Mesh] OR cannabis OR marijuana OR marihuana OR hash oil OR hashish. In 2014, when this review was established, specific searches were conducted using the appropriate MeSH terms for each topic area.

Once relevant literature is obtained, each finding is rated high, medium, or low quality based on the strengths and limitations of the methods which is determined by criteria in the GRADE system. The GRADE system is a well-established method for systematic literature review and has been used by the Cochrane Collaboration, British Medical Journal, American College of Physicians, World Health Organization, and many others [3]. Findings rated high quality are defined as "We are very confident that the true effect lies close to that of the estimate of the effect outlined in the study." These are well-designed and well-controlled studies with few limitations. Due to the fact that most studies included in our review are observational epidemiology studies, receiving a high quality rating does not necessarily imply causation. It simply implies that an observed association persists between an exposure and effect in an appropriately-sized study population after adjusting for appropriate confounders. Medium quality findings are defined as "we are moderately confident in the effect estimate outlined in the study. The true effect is likely to be close to the estimate of the effect, but there is a possibility that it is substantially different." For observational epidemiology studies this implies the finding of an observed association may be limited by a small study population or insufficient adjustment for important confounders. Low quality findings are defined as "our confidence in the effect estimate outlined in the study is limited. The true effect may be substantially different from the estimate of the effect." For observational epidemiology studies this implies the finding of an observed association with an interpretation that is significantly restricted by study limitations.

Findings from relevant literature are usually grouped based on outcome or the health effect in question. However, in some situations findings are further subdivided based on factors such as: age range of the exposed population, special subject circumstances such as pregnancy or breastfeeding, level or method of marijuana use, time period since last use of marijuana, amount of marijuana used, and THC concentration. Standardized definitions of level of marijuana use (daily, weekly, etc.) and age groups (child, adolescent, young adult, etc.) were established to help facilitate grouping of findings. Once findings are grouped appropriately, the evidence is drafted into evidence statements that summarize the quality and quantity of scientific evidence supporting an association between marijuana use and a health outcome.

3. Systematic review findings

In order to make our review findings easily interpretable we used a standardized rating system to classify evidence statements. These statements are also constructed to accurately portray the quality and quantity of all findings used to support the particular health outcome. Evidence statements all use standardized language from one of the following six classifications:

- Substantial evidence—indicates robust scientific findings that support an association between marijuana use and the outcome.

- Moderate evidence—indicates scientific findings that support an association, but these findings have some limitations.

- Limited evidence—indicates modest scientific findings that support an association, but these findings have significant limitations.

- Mixed evidence—indicates both supporting and opposing scientific findings for an association, with neither direction dominating.

- Insufficient evidence—indicates the outcome has not been sufficiently studied to conclude whether or not there is an association between marijuana use and the outcome.

- Body of research failing to show an association—indicates the topic has been researched without evidence of an association; is further classified as a limited, moderate, or substantial body of research.

In the following sections evidence statements will be discussed according to health topic and statements with enough findings to receive a substantial or moderate rating are displayed in tables. All statements, regardless of evidence level, are drafted by CDPHE technical staff, revised based on committee review and feedback from technical advisors and public stakeholders. Statements in their final form are approved by a vote of the committee.

3.1 Marijuana use among adolescents and young adults

The RMPHAC has reviewed the relationships between adolescent and young adult marijuana use on various areas of concern; including cognitive abilities, academic performance, mental health, and future substance use, displayed in **Table 1**. Specifically regarding cognitive and academic abilities, weekly marijuana use by adolescents is associated with deficits for at least twenty-eight days after last use. Weekly use among adolescents is also associated with failure to graduate from high school or complete a college degree. Information on how marijuana use affects short-term and long-term IQ is currently insufficient and limited, respectively. As with many of our statements that reflect long-term marijuana use, the paucity of long-term studies is a research gap that will hopefully improve due to the changing legal landscape of cannabis throughout the United States.

Adolescents and young adults who use marijuana are more likely to experience psychotic symptoms in adulthood (such as hallucinations, paranoia, and delusional beliefs), future psychotic disorders (such as schizophrenia), and suicidal thoughts or attempting suicide, when compared to adolescents and young adults who do not use marijuana. Additionally, those using marijuana with higher tetrahydrocannabinol (THC) concentration (>10% THC) are more likely than non-users to continue using and to develop future mental health symptoms and disorders. How marijuana use during adolescence affects symptoms or a diagnosis of anxiety in adulthood currently stands at a mixed evidence level, with fourteen articles contributing to this rating. Only one of which received a high quality rating and also reported mixed findings relevant to this evidence statement on anxiety [64]. Results from their main analysis did show an association with adolescent cannabis use and adulthood anxiety, however, results from a monozygotic-only co-twin control analysis reported no association [64].

Evidence shows that adolescents who use marijuana can develop cannabis use disorder, along with marijuana use being associated with developing use disorder for tobacco, alcohol, and other drugs. On a more positive note, evidence shows that adolescents who receive treatment for cannabis use disorder can decrease their use and dependence. Additionally, those who quit using marijuana have lower risks of adverse cognitive and mental health outcomes than those who continue to use.

3.2 Marijuana use and cancer

To assess how marijuana use may or may not be associated with cancer, the RMPHAC reviewed health effects of the chemicals released in marijuana smoke and vapor and evaluated how different rates of marijuana use relate to cancer. Strong evidence shows marijuana smoke contains many of the same cancer-causing chemicals found in tobacco smoke [109]. There is also substantial evidence that daily or near-daily marijuana smoking is associated with pre-malignant lesions in the airway.

	Substantial evidence	Moderate evidence
Benefits of quitting	Treatment for cannabis use disorder can reduce use and dependence [4–10]	Quitting or decreasing marijuana use lowers the risk of adverse mental health outcomes [11–14]
Cognitive and academic effects	Weekly, or more frequent, use is associated with a lower rate of graduating high school [15–23]	Weekly, or more frequent, use is associated with a lower rate of attaining a college degree (among those who start a degree program) [19, 24–29]
		Weekly, or more frequent, use is associated with ongoing cognitive and academic impairment for at least 28 days after last use [30–35]
Mental health	Daily or near daily use is associated with future psychotic disorders like schizophrenia [36–43]	Marijuana use is associated with suicidal thoughts or attempting suicide [22, 44–63]
	Use is associated with future psychotic symptoms (likelihood increases with more frequent use) [14, 40, 42, 64–80]	
Substance use, abuse, and addiction	Those who use marijuana can develop cannabis use disorder (addiction) [81–87]	Marijuana use is associated with future use and use disorder for alcohol [15, 20, 88–92]
	Marijuana use is associated with future use and use disorder for marijuana, tobacco and other drugs [13, 15, 20, 22, 25, 28, 79, 84, 87–105]	
High THC (%) concentration		Using marijuana with higher THC concentration (>10% THC) is associated with continued use [38, 106–108]
		Use of marijuana with higher THC concentration (>10% THC) is associated with future mental health symptoms and disorders [38, 78, 107]

Table 1.
Marijuana use among adolescents and young adults.

However, there is conflicting research for whether or not marijuana smoking is associated with lung cancer. As shown by the moderate evidence statement in **Table 2**, the body of research reviewed has failed to show an association between smoking less than the equivalent of one joint per day for 10 years and lung cancer.

Apart from the respiratory system, most of our statements are not in **Table 2** due to the limited evidence available concerning cancers of the bladder, prostate, head and neck. These limited statements all suggest these forms of cancer might not have any association with marijuana use. However, there is evidence that marijuana use among adult males may be associated with nonseminoma testicular cancer. High quality research on non-respiratory tract cancers related to marijuana use remains a research gap identified by the RMPHAC.

	Substantial evidence	Moderate evidence
Cancer and precancerous lesions	Daily or near daily use is associated with pre-cancerous lesions in airway [110–112]	Smoking less than the equivalent of one joint per day for 10 years is not associated with lung cancer [113–118]
Chemicals in MJ smoke or vapor	Marijuana smoke contains many of the same cancer causing chemicals as tobacco smoke [109, 119–122]	
Genitourinary Cancer		Use among adult males is associated with increased risk of nonseminoma testicular cancer [123–127]

Table 2.
Marijuana use and cancer.

Substantial evidence	Moderate evidence
	Marijuana users/consumers younger than 55 years of age are at an increased risk of stroke [128–145]

Table 3.
Marijuana use and cardiovascular effects.

3.3 Marijuana use and cardiovascular effects

Related to cardiovascular health effects, how marijuana use associates with myocardial infarction, stroke, and death from cardiovascular causes were reviewed. Evidence shows that marijuana use or consumption in those under the age of fifty-five years are at an increased risk of ischemic stoke, as shown in **Table 3**. However, currently there is only limited scientific evidence to support our statements on myocardial infarction and death related to a cardiovascular event.

3.4 Marijuana dose and drug interactions

An important metric to understand is how THC blood levels compare from various marijuana methods of use and the numerous concentrations of THC in available products on the retail marijuana market. For example, there is substantial evidence that smoking more than 10 mg THC (or 10–20% of a 1 g marijuana joint) produces a blood THC level near or above 5 ng/mL within 10 min. As we see the THC concentration of marijuana products increase, we can expect this association to remain strong. One important finding in **Table 4** is that it can take up to four hours after consuming an edible marijuana product to reach the peak THC blood concentration and feel the full effects. Another method of use, vaporized THC, shows moderate evidence of producing a similar blood THC level to smoking the same amount.

Within this topic the RMPHAC reviewed effects of secondhand marijuana smoke, drug-drug interactions involving marijuana, and relationships between marijuana and opioid use. There is credible evidence of clinically important drug-drug interactions between marijuana and multiple medications, including some anti-seizure medications and a common blood-thinner, warfarin. Data about potential interactions are

	Substantial evidence	Moderate evidence
THC blood levels resulting from different exposures	It takes up to four hours after ingesting marijuana (edible products) to reach peak blood THC levels [146–151]	Ingesting (edible products) more than 15 mg THC may produce a blood THC level above 5 ng/mL [148, 152–154]
	Smoking more than 10 mg THC produces a blood THC level near or above 5 ng/mL within 10 min [152, 155–159]	Inhaling vaporized THC produces a blood THC level similar to smoking the same dose [149, 159, 160]
Secondhand exposure	Typical secondhand marijuana smoke exposure is unlikely to cause a positive drug screen by urine or blood [161–169]	

Table 4.
Marijuana dose and drug interactions.

lacking for many drugs at this time and are likely to evolve substantially in the coming years. Other than our statement about secondhand marijuana smoke exposure being unlikely to cause a positive drug screen, our statements in this topic area are all based on limited evidence. Health effects resulting from secondhand marijuana smoke exposure is an area lacking in research. There is also conflicting evidence for whether or not marijuana use is associated with a decrease in opioid use among chronic pain patients or individuals with a history of problem drug use.

3.5 Marijuana use and driving

As with any psychoactive substance it is imperative to know how marijuana affects a person's ability to drive and the crash risks associated with use. To fully comprehend how marijuana causes driving impairment we must also understand the pharmacokinetics of THC in the human body to know how long these affects will persist after last use. **Table 5** displays all driving related statements that have evidence to provide a substantial or moderate rated statement. Current research shows substantial evidence that recent marijuana use by a driver increases the risk of a motor vehicle crash. In addition, using alcohol and marijuana together increases impairment and the risk of a motor vehicle crash more than using either substance alone.

The RMPHAC also set out to determine how various patterns of marijuana use affect driving. People that consume marijuana less-than-weekly are likely to experience impaired driving after using marijuana containing ten milligrams or more of THC. This statement holds true for smoking or consuming edible marijuana products. Research on driving impairment for those that consume more frequently than weekly is currently lacking in scientific literature. Due to this our evidence statement on crash risk for different levels of use (less-than-weekly compared to more frequent use) has received an insufficient rating at this time.

Articles measuring THC blood levels were also assessed to evaluate for any correlation to driving impairment, crash risk, and to develop statements informing consumers the amount of time to wait prior to driving. There is substantial evidence, including a randomized clinical trial [202], which has displayed meaningful driving impairment with a whole blood THC of 2–5 ng/mL. Additionally, moderate evidence points to a positive relationship between THC blood level and motor vehicle crash risk. In order for marijuana consumers to allow impairment to resolve, less-than-weekly consumers should wait at least six hours after smoking or

	Substantial evidence	Moderate evidence
Combined marijuana and alcohol use	Combined use of marijuana and alcohol increases crash risk more than either substance alone [170–181]	
Impairment and crash risk	Recent marijuana use/consumption by a driver increases the risk of a motor vehicle crash [170–172, 174, 182–188]	Higher THC blood level increases the risk of a motor vehicle crash [173, 178, 180, 189]
	Smoking more than 10 mg THC can lead to driving impairment [147, 155, 157, 177, 190–200]	Blood THC levels of impaired drivers are higher now than they were in the past [201]
	Orally ingesting more than 10 mg THC can lead driving impairment [146, 147, 153, 155]	
	Increased risk of driving impairment at blood THC as low as 2–5 ng/mL [155, 185, 190, 202–206]	
Time to wait before driving	Waiting at least 6 after smoking less than 18 mg allows driving impairment to resolve or nearly resolve [155, 190, 207]	Waiting at least 6 h after smoking about 35 mg allows driving impairment to resolve or nearly resolve [157, 192, 196]
	Waiting at least 8 h after orally ingesting less than 18 mg allows driving impairment to resolve or nearly resolve [147, 153, 155, 208]	

Table 5.
Marijuana use and driving.

eight hours after eating or drinking marijuana products. When consuming larger amounts of THC or for people that consume more frequently, evidence is currently insufficient to determine the safe amount of time for impairment to wear off. Evidence is also showing that blood THC levels of marijuana-impaired drivers are higher now than in the past, likely resulting from the increasing THC concentration of available marijuana products.

3.6 Marijuana use and gastrointestinal or reproductive effects

The RMPHAC reviewed how marijuana use may affect gastrointestinal disease, particularly cyclic vomiting, and infertility or abnormal reproductive function. Displayed in **Table 6**, evidence shows that long-time, daily or near daily marijuana use is associated with cyclic vomiting, also called cannabinoid hyperemesis syndrome (CHS). A majority of evidence supporting this statement is from case reports or case series of identified CHS patients, however, many review articles detail diagnostic criteria, treatment options, and the physiology behind marijuana use and CHS presentation [220]. Regarding reproductive function, there is limited research showing marijuana use is associated with male infertility or abnormal function, however, the research is conflicting for women.

3.7 Marijuana use and injury

The RMPHAC reviewed workplace, recreational and other non-driving injuries, burns from hash-oil extraction or failed electronic smoking devices, and physical

	Substantial evidence	Moderate evidence
Cyclic vomiting		Cyclic vomiting can occur with long-time, daily or near daily marijuana use/consumption (cannabinoid hyperemesis syndrome) [209–219]

Table 6.
Marijuana use and gastrointestinal and reproductive effects.

	Substantial evidence	Moderate evidence
Physical dating violence		Young adult women who use marijuana are unlikely to perpetrate physical dating violence [221–226]

Table 7.
Marijuana use and injury.

dating violence. Evidence shows mixed results for marijuana use affecting the risk of workplace injury, recreational injury, and other types of non-driving-related injury. There have been many reports of severe burns resulting from home-extraction of butane hash oil leading to explosions, and cases of electronic smoking devices exploding, leading to trauma and burns.

Concerning dating violence, **Table 7** shows our only statement reaching moderate or substantial levels of evidence is that young adult women who use marijuana are unlikely to perpetrate physical dating violence against their dating partners. Otherwise, evidence does show that young adults who use marijuana are unlikely to commit or be victims of physical dating violence, however evidence is limited at this time. Evidence for adolescent boys that use marijuana has mixed findings for physical dating violence perpetration and limited evidence for victimization, with evidence for adolescent girls being the opposite (**Table 7**).

3.8 Marijuana use and neurological, cognitive, and mental health effects

Similar to statements in our adolescent and young adult section, it is imperative to understand how marijuana could impact neurological, cognitive, and mental health in adult marijuana consumers. This section also explores how marijuana consumption relates to marijuana abuse and addiction among adult consumers. While our review on cognitive effects includes decision making, executive function, memory impairment, and lasting cognitive effects, strong evidence has been found only for memory impairment, as shown in **Table 8**. We have found substantial evidence that daily or near daily adult marijuana consumers are more likely than non-users to have memory impairments for at least seven days after last use. Evidence is mixed for whether or not these memory impairments or other cognitive effects last for at least twenty-eight days after last use, among the same population of adult consumers.

As with all psychoactive substances, mental health effects in adult marijuana consumers must be examined. An important acute effect of THC with substantial evidence is psychotic symptoms, such as hallucinations, paranoia, and delusional beliefs during intoxication, and these symptoms are worse with higher doses. Additionally, daily or near daily marijuana use is associated with developing a psychotic disorder such as schizophrenia. As detailed in our report focusing on the increasing concentration of THC in products available, there is increased public health concern as these

	Substantial evidence	Moderate evidence
Cognitive effects	Daily or near daily use is associated with impaired memory for at least 7 days [30, 227–235]	
Mental health effects	Use is associated with acute psychotic symptoms during intoxication, which are worse with higher doses [236–243]	
	Daily or near daily use is associated with future psychotic disorders like schizophrenia [38, 42, 107, 244–246]	Use of marijuana with THC concentration > 10% is associated with future psychotic disorders like schizophrenia [38, 107, 247]
Substance use, abuse and addiction	Those who use marijuana can develop cannabis use disorder (addiction) [82, 85, 86, 93, 248–252]	
	Treatment for cannabis use disorder can reduce use and dependence [4, 6, 8, 9, 253–257]	
	Those using daily or near daily can experience withdrawal symptoms when abstaining [11, 258–270]	

Table 8.
Marijuana use and neurological, cognitive, mental health effects.

products may lead to higher potential for adverse health effects in consumers [1]. This concern is substantiated by available research enabling us to provide a moderate rated statement showing association between higher concentration THC products and future psychotic disorders in adult marijuana consumers.

Finally, evidence shows marijuana consumers can experience withdrawal symptoms when abstaining and become addicted to marijuana or develop cannabis use disorder. However, as with adolescents, treatment for cannabis use disorder can reduce use and dependence in adult consumers. Many associations within this section lack high quality evidence or research currently exhibits mixed findings, such as marijuana use being associated with anxiety, depression, or bipolar disorder (**Table 8**).

3.9 Marijuana use during pregnancy and/or breastfeeding

Table 9 details our evidence concerning marijuana use during pregnancy and breastfeeding. Biological evidence shows THC passes through the placenta to the fetus and is present in the breast milk of women who use marijuana. Scientific evidence shows the fetus absorbs and metabolizes THC passed through the placenta and THC metabolites are found in the meconium or first stool passed by the newborn after birth. Additionally, infants who drink breast milk containing THC absorb and metabolize the THC. These statements show how important it is to understand how marijuana use during pregnancy and/or breastfeeding can affect the offspring or impact delivery of the offspring.

Specifically regarding exposed offspring, the RMPHAC reviews potential effects starting at birth and later in childhood or adolescence. Marijuana use during pregnancy has shown to not be associated with birth defects in general, but limited evidence of an association with an increased risk of heart defects, stillbirth, and decreased growth in offspring. Stronger evidence was found for effects that are seen

	Substantial evidence	Moderate evidence
Effects on exposed offspring		Prenatal marijuana exposure is associated with reduced cognitive function, academic ability, and IQ scores in childhood [271–280]
		Prenatal marijuana exposure is associated with attention problems in childhood [273, 281–285]
Birth defects		Prenatal marijuana use is not associated with birth defects [286–292]
Preterm delivery or abnormal birth weight		Maternal use during pregnancy is associated with infants being born small for gestational age (birth weight less than 10th percentile for gestational age) [286, 287, 289, 292–305]
Biological evidence concerning marijuana use during pregnancy and breastfeeding		
THC is passed through the placenta of women who use marijuana, the fetus absorbs and metabolizes the THC, and THC metabolites are found in the meconium [306–310].		
THC is present in the breast milk of women who use marijuana. Infants who drink breast milk containing THC absorb and metabolize the THC [311–316].		

Table 9.
Marijuana use during pregnancy and/or breastfeeding.

in offspring years after birth if a child's mother used marijuana while pregnant. These include impaired cognitive function and academic ability, lower IQ scores, and attention problems in childhood.

3.10 Marijuana use and respiratory effects

While consumers have a variety of marijuana products to choose from, smoking marijuana flower remains the most common method of use and thus respiratory effects must be evaluated [317]. The RMPHAC reviews respiratory diseases such as chronic obstructive pulmonary disorder (COPD), chronic bronchitis and asthma, respiratory infections, lung function relative to smoked marijuana. The committee has also reviewed potential health effects of vaporized marijuana as those products have emerged on the legal market. Displayed in **Table 10**, strong evidence shows an association between daily or near-daily marijuana use and chronic bronchitis, including chronic cough, sputum production, and wheezing. Weaker evidence shows daily or near-daily marijuana use may be associated with bullous lung disease leading to pneumothorax in individuals younger than forty years of age. Additionally, limited evidence does show frequent smokers who switch from marijuana smoking to marijuana vaporizing may have fewer respiratory symptoms and improved pulmonary function. Finally, a notable effect of acute marijuana smoking is a short-term improvement in lung airflow, though evidence contributing to this statement is dated (**Table 10**).

3.11 Unintentional marijuana exposure in children

As marijuana becomes more accessible to the public, we must consider unintentional exposures in homes with children and how packaging can affect these. Strong evidence was found, shown in **Table 11**, that more unintentional exposures of children occur in states with increased legal access to marijuana, and exposures can lead

	Substantial evidence	**Moderate evidence**
Smoked marijuana	Use is associated with chronic bronchitis with cough, wheezing and mucus [318–327]	
	Acute use is associated with short-term lung airflow improvement [328–330]	

Table 10.
Marijuana use and respiratory effects.

Substantial evidence	**Moderate evidence**
Legal marijuana access increases unintentional marijuana exposures in children [331–341]	Child-resistant packaging reduces unintentional pediatric poisonings [342–344]

Table 11.
Unintentional marijuana exposure in children.

to significant clinical effects requiring medical attention and even hospitalization. However, evidence does show that child-resistant packaging reduces unintentional pediatric marijuana poisonings (**Table 11**).

4. Public health statements and recommendations

Once evidence statements have been drafted and approved by the RMPHAC, the next step (number 6 from our systematic review process) is to translate the evidence into public health statements. These are designed to accurately reflect the evidence statements using language the public can understand. The committee also wanted to ensure these statements conveyed the volume and quality of research related to the outcome and allowed the statement to stand on its own without context. Similar to our evidence statements, these use standardized language to represent the strength of relationship and use the phrase "associated with" to represent epidemiologic associations that do not imply causation. As of the date of this book's publication CDPHE has seventy-four public health statements corresponding to all our evidence statements rated moderate or substantial.

In a similar manner, public health statements are subsequently drafted into public health recommendations. These are synthesized in order to inform the development of evidence-based prevention and education campaigns performed by CDPHE. Furthermore, recommendations are separated by data quality issues, surveillance, and education. Our recommendations share common themes to those put forth by the National Academies of Sciences, Engineering, and Medicine's review of health effects associated with cannabis and cannabinoids [345].

Data quality issues are defined as recommendations to improve current data collection deficiencies at the clinical or governmental level that prevent full analysis of public health outcomes related to marijuana use. It is especially important to improve data quality by systematically collecting information on the frequency, amount, THC content, and method of marijuana use in both public health surveillance and medical care settings. Clinicians should routinely screen for marijuana use during hospitalizations, especially among pregnant or adolescent patients.

Public health surveillance recommendations are based on improving capacity to detect an acute public health danger (e.g., real time emergency department surveillance to detect poisonings from contaminated product); the ability to characterize chronic public health dangers to support policy and other intervention decisions; or the ability to generate epidemiologic data to contribute to planning and evaluating population level interventions. Questions regarding marijuana use should be continued on population-based surveys such as the Behavioral Risk Factor Surveillance System, the Healthy Kids Colorado Survey, and Pregnancy Risk Assessment Monitoring System. Additionally, methods should be expanded to collect more detailed information, such as quantity and methods of use, THC content of products used, and adverse effects experienced.

Education recommendations are included to ensure evidence-based information on potential health effects of marijuana use is provided to the appropriate target audiences. Public education is especially important related to the effects of use during pregnancy, adolescent use, driving after use, increasing THC concentration of products, and unsafe storage around children. Education for health care providers should also be emphasized on the need for marijuana use screening, the known health effects of use, and encouraging more open dialog between providers and patients.

5. Research gaps

In addition to public health recommendations, important research gaps related to the population-based health effects of marijuana use were identified during the literature review process. These research gaps are based on common limitations of existing research or issues important to public education or policymaking. Research gaps particularly important to public health and safety include the need for: (1) research on the effects of marijuana use on pregnant women and their offspring, including while breastfeeding; (2) research on marijuana and marijuana products that contain THC concentrations consistent with products currently available in legalized markets; (3) research on health effects among individuals who have used marijuana frequently for a long period of time; (4) research on driving impairment among people who use marijuana more than weekly and may have developed tolerance; (5) research to better characterize the pharmacokinetics/pharmacodynamics, potential drug interactions, health effects, and impairment related to non-smoking methods of marijuana use such as edible products and vaporizing; and (6) research to better describe the risk of adverse health effects due to contamination of the marijuana product by fungi, mold, solvents, additives, heavy metals, and pesticides.

Other research gaps identify areas that need improvement in new research moving forward. Such as studies using better and more standardized indicators of marijuana use, including frequency, THC content, and route of exposure, including populations that use marijuana daily or near daily, and stratifying groups by age and gender. Finally one step to provide strong evidence would be research data on a community based cohort to study both beneficial and adverse health effects of marijuana consumption. Identifying these research gaps provides researchers and funding sources with an important framework to prioritize areas of research related to marijuana use and public health.

6. Conclusion

Since 2014, when CDPHE was designated to monitor the emerging science and medical information relevant to the health effects associated with marijuana use, the

RMPHAC and CDPHE technical staff have conducted an ongoing systematic review of scientific literature to establish over one hundred evidence statements with eleven health topics. Our mission is to translate the science into meaningful public health statements and recommendations to inform and educate the general public, healthcare providers, and everyone in-between on the health effects associated with marijuana use.

First, the committee established a strict process to ensure a thorough and unbiased review, set up quarterly meetings to enable open discussions on a continuous basis, and come to consensus on the science and how to present this information to the public. After establishing our process, evidence from scientific research is constantly reviewed and added when appropriate to form a comprehensive review of marijuana health effects across eleven health topic. Strong evidence statements from all health topics were displayed in tables and key findings were detailed in subsections to provide an overview of effects associated with marijuana use across many different populations and health topics. Additional details were described on how these evidence statements are used to inform public health policy in the State of Colorado through public health recommendations and research gaps.

Acknowledgements

Elyse Contreras, DeLayna Goulding, Daniel I. Vigil, Katelyn E. Hall, Michael Van Dyke, Shireen Banerji, Russell Bowler, Ashley Brooks-Russell, Christopher Domen, Heather Krug, David J Kroll, Sharon Langendoerfer, Andrew Monte, Kenneth Novoa, Judith Shlay, Elizabeth Stuyt, George Sam Wang, Bernadette Albanese, Lisa Barker, Laura Borgelt, Alvin C. Bronstein, Todd Carlson, Rowena Crow, Teresa Foo, Ken Gershman, Tista Ghosh, Heath Harmon, Rebecca Helfand, Renee M. Johnson, Bruce Mendelson, Madeline Morris, Kristina T. Phillips, Allison Rosenthal, Kim Siegal, Scott Simpson, Christian Thurstone.

Conflict of interest

"The authors declare no conflict of interest."

Author details

Richard Holdman
Colorado Department of Public Health and Environment, Denver, United States

*Address all correspondence to: richard.holdman@state.co.us

References

[1] Monitoring Health Concerns Related to Maijuana; Reports and Summaries. Colorado Department of Public Health and Environment. Colorado Department of Public Health and Environment. 2022. Available from: https://marijuanahealthinfo.colorado.gov/reports-and-summaries

[2] Moher D, Liberati A, Tetzlaff J, Altman DG, Group P. Preferred reporting items for systematic reviews and meta-analyses: the PRISMA statement. Journal of Clinical Epidemiology. 2009;**62**(10):1006-1012

[3] GRADE guidelines—best practices using the GRADE framework.: GRADE working group; 2014. Available from: http://training.cochrane.org/path/grade-approach-evaluating-quality-evidence-pathway

[4] Dennis M, Godley SH, Diamond G, Tims FM, Babor T, Donaldson J, et al. The Cannabis Youth Treatment (CYT) Study: Main findings from two randomized trials. Journal of Substance Abuse Treatment. 2004;**27**(3):197-213

[5] Hendriks V, van der Schee E, Blanken P. Treatment of adolescents with a cannabis use disorder: Main findings of a randomized controlled trial comparing multidimensional family therapy and cognitive behavioral therapy in The Netherlands. Drug and Alcohol Dependence. 2011;**119**(1-2):64-71

[6] Olmos A, Tirado-Munoz J, Farre M, Torrens M. The efficacy of computerized interventions to reduce cannabis use: A systematic review and meta-analysis. Addictive Behaviors. 2018;**79**:52-60

[7] Rigter H, Henderson CE, Pelc I, Tossmann P, Phan O, Hendriks V, et al. Multidimensional family therapy lowers the rate of cannabis dependence in adolescents: A randomised controlled trial in Western European outpatient settings. Drug and Alcohol Dependence. 2013;**130**(1-3):85-93

[8] Stanger C, Budney AJ, Kamon JL, Thostensen J. A randomized trial of contingency management for adolescent marijuana abuse and dependence. Drug and Alcohol Dependence. 2009;**105**(3):240-247

[9] Stanger C, Ryan SR, Scherer EA, Norton GE, Budney AJ. Clinic- and home-based contingency management plus parent training for adolescent cannabis use disorders. Journal of the American Academy of Child and Adolescent Psychiatry. 2015;**54**(6):445-53 e2

[10] Stanger C, Scherer EA, Babbin SF, Ryan SR, Budney AJ. Abstinence based incentives plus parent training for adolescent alcohol and other substance misuse. Psychology of Addictive Behaviors. 2017;**31**(4):385-392

[11] Jacobus J, Squeglia LM, Escobar S, McKenna BM, Hernandez MM, Bagot KS, et al. Changes in marijuana use symptoms and emotional functioning over 28-days of monitored abstinence in adolescent marijuana users. Psychopharmacology. 2017;**234**(23-24):3431-3442

[12] Pahl K, Brook JS, Koppel J. Trajectories of marijuana use and psychological adjustment among urban African American and Puerto Rican women. Psychological Medicine. 2011;**41**(8):1775-1783

[13] Swift W, Coffey C, Carlin JB, Degenhardt L, Patton GC. Adolescent cannabis users at 24 years: Trajectories to regular weekly use and dependence in young adulthood. Addiction. 2008;**103**(8):1361-1370

[14] van Gastel WA, Vreeker A, Schubart CD, MacCabe JH, Kahn RS, Boks MP. Change in cannabis use in the general population: A longitudinal study on the impact on psychotic experiences. Schizophrenia Research. 2014;**157**(1-3):266-270

[15] Brook JS, Balka EB, Whiteman M. The risks for late adolescence of early adolescent marijuana use. American Journal of Public Health. 1999;**89**(10):1549-1554

[16] Ehrenreich H, Nahapetyan L, Orpinas P, Song X. Marijuana use from middle to high school: Co-occurring problem behaviors, teacher-rated academic skills and sixth-grade predictors. Journal of Youth and Adolescence. 2015;**44**(10):1929-1940

[17] Fergusson DM, Horwood LJ, Beautrais AL. Cannabis and educational achievement. Addiction. 2003;**98**(12):1681-1692

[18] Green KM, Doherty EE, Ensminger ME. Long-term consequences of adolescent cannabis use: Examining intermediary processes. The American Journal of Drug and Alcohol Abuse. 2017;**43**(5):567-575

[19] Horwood LJ, Fergusson DM, Hayatbakhsh MR, Najman JM, Coffey C, Patton GC, et al. Cannabis use and educational achievement: Findings from three Australasian cohort studies. Drug and Alcohol Dependence. 2010;**110**(3):247-253

[20] Lynne-Landsman SD, Bradshaw CP, Ialongo NS. Testing a developmental cascade model of adolescent substance use trajectories and young adult adjustment. Development and Psychopathology. 2010;**22**(4):933-948

[21] Melchior M, Bolze C, Fombonne E, Surkan PJ, Pryor L, Jauffret-Roustide M. Early cannabis initiation and educational attainment: Is the association causal? Data from the French TEMPO study. International Journal of Epidemiology. 2017;**46**(5):1641-1650

[22] Silins E, Horwood LJ, Patton GC, Fergusson DM, Olsson CA, Hutchinson DM, et al. Young adult sequelae of adolescent cannabis use: An integrative analysis. Lancet Psychiatry. 2014;**1**(4):286-293

[23] Stiby AI, Hickman M, Munafo MR, Heron J, Yip VL, Macleod J. Adolescent cannabis and tobacco use and educational outcomes at age 16: Birth cohort study. Addiction. 2015;**110**(4):658-668

[24] Baggio S, Iglesias K, Deline S, Studer J, Henchoz Y, Mohler-Kuo M, et al. Not in education, employment, or training status among young Swiss men. Longitudinal associations with mental health and substance use. The Journal of Adolescent Health. 2015;**56**(2):238-243

[25] Fergusson DM, Horwood LJ. Does cannabis use encourage other forms of illicit drug use? Addiction. 2000;**95**(4):505-520

[26] Fergusson DM, Boden JM. Cannabis use and later life outcomes. Addiction. 2008;**103**(6):969-976; discussion 77-8

[27] Patrick ME, Schulenberg JE, O'Malley PM. High school substance use as a predictor of college attendance, completion, and dropout: A national multi-cohort longitudinal study. Youth Society. 2016;**48**(3):425-447

[28] Schaefer JD, Hamdi NR, Malone SM, Vrieze S, Wilson S, McGue M, et al. Associations between adolescent cannabis use and young-adult functioning in three longitudinal twin studies. Proceedings of the National Academy of Sciences of the United States of America. 2021;**118**(14):e2013180118

[29] Wilhite ER, Ashenhurst JR, Marino EN, Fromme K. Freshman year alcohol and marijuana use prospectively predict time to college graduation and subsequent adult roles and independence. Journal of American College Health. 2017;**65**(6):413-422

[30] Bolla KI, Brown K, Eldreth D, Tate K, Cadet JL. Dose-related neurocognitive effects of marijuana use. Neurology. 2002;**59**(9):1337-1343

[31] Hooper SR, Woolley D, De Bellis MD. Intellectual, neurocognitive, and academic achievement in abstinent adolescents with cannabis use disorder. Psychopharmacology. 2014;**231**(8):1467-1477

[32] Medina KL, Hanson KL, Schweinsburg AD, Cohen-Zion M, Nagel BJ, Tapert SF. Neuropsychological functioning in adolescent marijuana users: Subtle deficits detectable after a month of abstinence. Journal of the International Neuropsychological Society. 2007;**13**(5):807-820

[33] Pope HG Jr, Gruber AJ, Hudson JI, Cohane G, Huestis MA, Yurgelun-Todd D. Early-onset cannabis use and cognitive deficits: What is the nature of the association? Drug and Alcohol Dependence. 2003;**69**(3):303-310

[34] Scott JC, Slomiak ST, Jones JD, Rosen AFG, Moore TM, Gur RC. Association of cannabis with cognitive functioning in adolescents and young adults: A systematic review and meta-analysis. JAMA Psychiatry. 2018;**75**(6):585-595

[35] Selamoglu A, Langley C, Crean R, Savulich G, Cormack F, Sahakian BJ, et al. Neuropsychological performance in young adults with cannabis use disorder. Journal of Psychopharmacology. 2021;**35**(11):1349-1355

[36] Arranz S, Monferrer N, Jose Algora M, Cabezas A, Sole M, Vilella E, et al. The relationship between the level of exposure to stress factors and cannabis in recent onset psychosis. Schizophrenia Research. 2018;**201**:352-359

[37] Bechtold J, Simpson T, White HR, Pardini D. Chronic adolescent marijuana use as a risk factor for physical and mental health problems in young adult men. Psychology of Addictive Behaviors. 2015;**29**(3):552-563

[38] Di Forti M, Marconi A, Carra E, Fraietta S, Trotta A, Bonomo M, et al. Proportion of patients in south London with first-episode psychosis attributable to use of high potency cannabis: A case-control study. Lancet Psychiatry. 2015;**2**(3):233-238

[39] Godin SL, Shehata S. Adolescent cannabis use and later development of schizophrenia: An updated systematic review of longitudinal studies. Journal of Clinical Psychology. 2022;**78**(7):1331-1340

[40] Marconi A, Di Forti M, Lewis CM, Murray RM, Vassos E. Meta-analysis of the association between the level of cannabis use and risk of psychosis. Schizophrenia Bulletin. 2016;**42**(5):1262-1269

[41] Mustonen A, Niemela S, Nordstrom T, Murray GK, Maki P, Jaaskelainen E, et al. Adolescent cannabis use, baseline prodromal symptoms and

the risk of psychosis. The British Journal of Psychiatry. 2018;**212**(4):227-233

[42] van Os J, Bak M, Hanssen M, Bijl RV, de Graaf R, Verdoux H. Cannabis use and psychosis: A longitudinal population-based study. American Journal of Epidemiology. 2002;**156**(4):319-327

[43] Zammit S, Allebeck P, Andreasson S, Lundberg I, Lewis G. Self reported cannabis use as a risk factor for schizophrenia in Swedish conscripts of 1969: Historical cohort study. BMJ. 2002;**325**(7374):1199

[44] Agrawal A, Tillman R, Grucza RA, Nelson EC, McCutcheon VV, Few L, et al. Reciprocal relationships between substance use and disorders and suicidal ideation and suicide attempts in the Collaborative Study of the Genetics of Alcoholism. Journal of Affective Disorders. 2017;**213**:96-104

[45] Alexander D, Niemelä S, Scott JG, Salom C, Emily H, Miettunen J, et al. Does cannabis use in adolescence predict self-harm or suicide? Results from a Finnish Birth-Cohort Study. Acta Psychiatrica Scandinavica. 2021;**145**(3):234-243

[46] Borges G, Bagge CL, Orozco R. A literature review and meta-analyses of cannabis use and suicidality. Journal of Affective Disorders. 2016;**195**:63-74

[47] Borges G, Benjet C, Orozco R, Medina-Mora ME, Menendez D. Alcohol, cannabis and other drugs and subsequent suicide ideation and attempt among young Mexicans. Journal of Psychiatric Research. 2017;**91**:74-82

[48] Buckner JD, Lemke AW, Walukevich KA. Cannabis use and suicidal ideation: Test of the utility of the interpersonal-psychological theory of suicide. Psychiatry Research. 2017;**253**:256-259

[49] Sellers CM, Diaz-Valdes Iriarte A, Wyman Battalen A, O'Brien KHM. Alcohol and marijuana use as daily predictors of suicide ideation and attempts among adolescents prior to psychiatric hospitalization. Psychiatry Research. 2019;**273**:672-677

[50] Consoli A, Peyre H, Speranza M, Hassler C, Falissard B, Touchette E, et al. Suicidal behaviors in depressed adolescents: Role of perceived relationships in the family. Child and Adolescent Psychiatry and Mental Health. 2013;**7**(1):8

[51] Gobbi G, Atkin T, Zytynski T, Wang S, Askari S, Boruff J, et al. Association of cannabis use in adolescence and risk of depression, anxiety, and suicidality in young adulthood: A systematic review and meta-analysis. JAMA Psychiatry. 2019;**76**(4):426-434

[52] Gukasyan N, Strain EC. Relationship between cannabis use frequency and major depressive disorder in adolescents: Findings from the National Survey on Drug Use and Health 2012-2017. Drug and Alcohol Dependence. 2020;**208**:107867

[53] Guo L, Wang W, Du X, Guo Y, Li W, Zhao M, et al. Associations of substance use behaviors with suicidal ideation and suicide attempts among US and Chinese adolescents. Frontiers in Psychiatry. 2020;**11**:611579

[54] Han B, Compton WM, Einstein EB, Volkow ND. Associations of suicidality trends with cannabis use as a function of sex and depression status. JAMA Network Open. 2021;**4**(6):e2113025

[55] Hengartner MP, Angst J, Ajdacic-Gross V, Rossler W. Cannabis use

during adolescence and the occurrence of depression, suicidality and anxiety disorder across adulthood: Findings from a longitudinal cohort study over 30 years. Journal of Affective Disorders. 2020;**272**:98-103

[56] Kokkevi A, Richardson C, Olszewski D, Matias J, Monshouwer K, Bjarnason T. Multiple substance use and self-reported suicide attempts by adolescents in 16 European countries. European Child & Adolescent Psychiatry. 2012;**21**(8):443-450

[57] Labuhn M, LaBore K, Ahmed T, Ahmed R. Trends and instigators among young adolescent suicide in the United States. Public Health. 2021;**199**:51-56

[58] Pereira-Morales AJ, Adan A, Camargo A, Forero DA. Substance use and suicide risk in a sample of young Colombian adults: An exploration of psychosocial factors. The American Journal on Addictions. 2017;**26**(4):388-394

[59] Rasic D, Weerasinghe S, Asbridge M, Langille DB. Longitudinal associations of cannabis and illicit drug use with depression, suicidal ideation and suicidal attempts among Nova Scotia high school students. Drug and Alcohol Dependence. 2013;**129**(1-2):49-53

[60] Sampasa-Kanyinga H, Dupuis LC, Ray R. Prevalence and correlates of suicidal ideation and attempts among children and adolescents. International Journal of Adolescent Medicine and Health. 2017;**29**(2):/j/ijamh.2017.29.issue-2/ijamh-2015-0053/ijamh-2015-0053.xml

[61] Spears M, Montgomery AA, Gunnell D, Araya R. Factors associated with the development of self-harm amongst a socio-economically deprived cohort of adolescents in Santiago, Chile. Social Psychiatry and Psychiatric Epidemiology. 2014;**49**(4):629-637

[62] Weeks M, Colman I. Predictors of suicidal behaviors in canadian adolescents with no recent history of depression. Archives of Suicide Research. 2017;**21**(2):354-364

[63] Zhang X, Wu LT. Suicidal ideation and substance use among adolescents and young adults: A bidirectional relation? Drug and Alcohol Dependence. 2014;**142**:63-73

[64] Schaefer JD, Jang SK, Vrieze S, Iacono WG, McGue M, Wilson S. Adolescent cannabis use and adult psychoticism: A longitudinal co-twin control analysis using data from two cohorts. Journal of Abnormal Psychology. 2021;**130**(7):691-701

[65] Albertella L, Le Pelley ME, Copeland J. Cannabis use in early adolescence is associated with higher negative schizotypy in females. European Psychiatry. 2017;**45**:235-241

[66] Albertella L, Le Pelley ME, Yucel M, Copeland J. Age moderates the association between frequent cannabis use and negative schizotypy over time. Addictive Behaviors. 2018;**87**:183-189

[67] Arseneault L, Cannon M, Witton J, Murray RM. Causal association between cannabis and psychosis: Examination of the evidence. The British Journal of Psychiatry. 2004;**184**:110-117

[68] Bourque J, Afzali MH, O'Leary-Barrett M, Conrod P. Cannabis use and psychotic-like experiences trajectories during early adolescence: The coevolution and potential mediators. Journal of Child Psychology and Psychiatry. 2017;**58**(12):1360-1369

[69] Carlyle M, Constable T, Walter ZC, Wilson J, Newland G, Hides L. Cannabis-induced dysphoria/paranoia mediates the link between childhood trauma and psychotic-like experiences in young cannabis users. Schizophrenia Research. 2021;**238**:178-184

[70] Fergusson DM, Horwood LJ, Ridder EM. Tests of causal linkages between cannabis use and psychotic symptoms. Addiction. 2005;**100**(3):354-366

[71] Henquet C, Krabbendam L, Spauwen J, Kaplan C, Lieb R, Wittchen HU, et al. Prospective cohort study of cannabis use, predisposition for psychosis, and psychotic symptoms in young people. BMJ. 2005;**330**(7481):11

[72] Jones HJ, Gage SH, Heron J, Hickman M, Lewis G, Munafo MR, et al. Association of combined patterns of tobacco and cannabis use in adolescence with psychotic experiences. JAMA Psychiatry. 2018;**75**(3):240-246

[73] Kiburi SK, Molebatsi K, Ntlantsana V, Lynskey MT. Cannabis use in adolescence and risk of psychosis: Are there factors that moderate this relationship? A systematic review and meta-analysis. Substance Abuse. 2021:**42**(4)527-542

[74] Kuepper R, van Os J, Lieb R, Wittchen HU, Hofler M, Henquet C. Continued cannabis use and risk of incidence and persistence of psychotic symptoms: 10 year follow-up cohort study. BMJ. 2011;**342**:d738

[75] Leadbeater BJ, Ames ME, Linden-Carmichael AN. Age-varying effects of cannabis use frequency and disorder on symptoms of psychosis, depression and anxiety in adolescents and adults. Addiction. 2019;**114**(2):278-293

[76] McGrath J, Welham J, Scott J, Varghese D, Degenhardt L, Hayatbakhsh MR, et al. Association between cannabis use and psychosis-related outcomes using sibling pair analysis in a cohort of young adults. Archives of General Psychiatry. 2010;**67**(5):440-447

[77] Pardo M, Matali JL, Sivoli J, Regina VB, Butjosa A, Dolz M, et al. Early onset psychosis and cannabis use: Prevalence, clinical presentation and influence of daily use. Asian Journal of Psychiatry. 2021;**62**:102714

[78] Quattrone D, Ferraro L, Tripoli G, La Cascia C, Quigley H, Quattrone A, et al. Daily use of high-potency cannabis is associated with more positive symptoms in first-episode psychosis patients: The EU-GEI case-control study. Psychological Medicine. 2020:**51**(8)1-9

[79] Shanahan L, Steinhoff A, Bechtiger L, Copeland WE, Ribeaud D, Eisner M, et al. Frequent teenage cannabis use: Prevalence across adolescence and associations with young adult psychopathology and functional well-being in an urban cohort. Drug and Alcohol Dependence. 2021;**228**:109063

[80] Wainberg M, Jacobs GR, di Forti M, Tripathy SJ. Cannabis, schizophrenia genetic risk, and psychotic experiences: A cross-sectional study of 109,308 participants from the UK Biobank. Translational Psychiatry. 2021;**11**(1):211

[81] Forman-Hoffman VL, Glasheen C, Batts KR. Marijuana use, recent marijuana initiation, and progression to marijuana use disorder among young male and female adolescents aged 12-14 living in US Households. Substance Abuse. 2017;**11**:1178221817711159

[82] Hasin DS, Saha TD, Kerridge BT, Goldstein RB, Chou SP, Zhang H, et al.

Prevalence of marijuana use disorders in the United States between 2001-2002 and 2012-2013. JAMA Psychiatry. 2015;**72**(12):1235-1242

[83] Marel C, Sunderland M, Mills KL, Slade T, Teesson M, Chapman C. Conditional probabilities of substance use disorders and associated risk factors: Progression from first use to use disorder on alcohol, cannabis, stimulants, sedatives and opioids. Drug and Alcohol Dependence. 2019;**194**:136-142

[84] Millar SR, Mongan D, Smyth BP, Perry IJ, Galvin B. Relationships between age at first substance use and persistence of cannabis use and cannabis use disorder. BMC Public Health. 2021;**21**(1):997

[85] Richter L, Pugh BS, Ball SA. Assessing the risk of marijuana use disorder among adolescents and adults who use marijuana. The American Journal of Drug and Alcohol Abuse. 2017;**43**(3):247-260

[86] Schuermeyer J, Salomonsen-Sautel S, Price RK, Balan S, Thurstone C, Min SJ, et al. Temporal trends in marijuana attitudes, availability and use in Colorado compared to non-medical marijuana states: 2003-11. Drug and Alcohol Dependence. 2014;**140**:145-155

[87] Simpson KA, Cho J, Barrington-Trimis JL. The association of type of cannabis product used and frequency of use with problematic cannabis use in a sample of young adult cannabis users. Drug and Alcohol Dependence. 2021;**226**:108865

[88] Guttmannova K, Kosterman R, White HR, Bailey JA, Lee JO, Epstein M, et al. The association between regular marijuana use and adult mental health outcomes. Drug and Alcohol Dependence. 2017;**179**:109-116

[89] Otten R, Mun CJ, Dishion TJ. The social exigencies of the gateway progression to the use of illicit drugs from adolescence into adulthood. Addictive Behaviors. 2017;**73**:144-150

[90] Silins E, Swift W, Slade T, Toson B, Rodgers B, Hutchinson DM. A prospective study of the substance use and mental health outcomes of young adult former and current cannabis users. Drug and Alcohol Review. 2017;**36**(5):618-625

[91] Swift W, Coffey C, Degenhardt L, Carlin JB, Romaniuk H, Patton GC. Cannabis and progression to other substance use in young adults: Findings from a 13-year prospective population-based study. Journal of Epidemiology and Community Health. 2012;**66**(7):e26

[92] Taylor M, Collin SM, Munafo MR, MacLeod J, Hickman M, Heron J. Patterns of cannabis use during adolescence and their association with harmful substance use behaviour: Findings from a UK birth cohort. Journal of Epidemiology and Community Health. 2017;**71**(8):764-770

[93] Feingold D, Livne O, Rehm J, Lev-Ran S. Probability and correlates of transition from cannabis use to DSM-5 cannabis use disorder: Results from a large-scale nationally representative study. Drug and Alcohol Review. 2020;**39**(2):142-151

[94] Lanza HI, Bello MS, Cho J, Barrington-Trimis JL, McConnell R, Braymiller JL, et al. Tobacco and cannabis poly-substance and poly-product use trajectories across adolescence and young adulthood. Preventive Medicine. 2021;**148**:106545

[95] Copeland WE, Hill SN, Shanahan L. Adult psychiatric, substance, and functional outcomes of different

definitions of early cannabis use. Journal of the American Academy of Child and Adolescent Psychiatry. 2021;**61**(4):533-543

[96] Fergusson DM, Boden JM, Horwood LJ. Cannabis use and other illicit drug use: Testing the cannabis gateway hypothesis. Addiction. 2006;**101**(4):556-569

[97] Fiellin LE, Tetrault JM, Becker WC, Fiellin DA, Hoff RA. Previous use of alcohol, cigarettes, and marijuana and subsequent abuse of prescription opioids in young adults. The Journal of Adolescent Health. 2013;**52**(2):158-163

[98] Moss HB, Chen CM, Yi HY. Early adolescent patterns of alcohol, cigarettes, and marijuana polysubstance use and young adult substance use outcomes in a nationally representative sample. Drug and Alcohol Dependence. 2014;**136**:51-62

[99] Nakawaki B, Crano WD. Predicting adolescents' persistence, non-persistence, and recent onset of nonmedical use of opioids and stimulants. Addictive Behaviors. 2012;**37**(6):716-721

[100] Schepis TS, Krishnan-Sarin S. Characterizing adolescent prescription misusers: A population-based study. Journal of the American Academy of Child and Adolescent Psychiatry. 2008;**47**(7):745-754

[101] Zaman T, Malowney M, Knight J, Boyd JW. Co-occurrence of substance-related and other mental health disorders among adolescent cannabis users. Journal of Addiction Medicine. 2015;**9**(4):317-321

[102] Berg CJ, Haardörfer R, Lanier A, Childs D, Foster B, Getachew B, et al. Tobacco use trajectories in young adults: Analyses of predictors across systems levels. Nicotine & Tobacco Research. 2020;**22**(11):2075-2084

[103] Cornacchione Ross J, Sutfin EL, Suerken C, Walker S, Wolfson M, Reboussin BA. Longitudinal associations between marijuana and cigar use in young adults. Drug and Alcohol Dependence. 2020;**211**:107964

[104] Mayer ME, Kong G, Barrington-Trimis JL, McConnell R, Leventhal AM, Krishnan-Sarin S. Blunt and non-blunt cannabis use and risk of subsequent combustible tobacco product use among adolescents. Nicotine & Tobacco Research. 2020;**22**(8):1409-1413

[105] Rubinstein ML, Rait MA, Prochaska JJ. Frequent marijuana use is associated with greater nicotine addiction in adolescent smokers. Drug and Alcohol Dependence. 2014;**141**:159-162

[106] Barrington-Trimis JL, Cho J, Ewusi-Boisvert E, Hasin D, Unger JB, Miech RA, et al. Risk of persistence and progression of use of 5 cannabis products after experimentation among adolescents. JAMA Network Open. 2020;**3**(1):e1919792

[107] Di Forti M, Quattrone D, Freeman TP, Tripoli G, Gayer-Anderson C, Quigley H, et al. The contribution of cannabis use to variation in the incidence of psychotic disorder across Europe (EU-GEI): A multicentre case-control study. Lancet Psychiatry. 2019;**6**(5):427-436

[108] Hines LA, Freeman TP, Gage SH, Zammit S, Hickman M, Cannon M, et al. Association of high-potency cannabis use with mental health and substance use in adolescence. JAMA Psychiatry. 2020;**77**(10):1044-1051

[109] Moir D, Rickert WS, Levasseur G, Larose Y, Maertens R, White P, et al. A comparison of mainstream and sidestream marijuana

and tobacco cigarette smoke produced under two machine smoking conditions. Chemical Research in Toxicology. 2008;**21**(2):494-502

[110] Barsky SH, Roth MD, Kleerup EC, Simmons M, Tashkin DP. Histopathologic and molecular alterations in bronchial epithelium in habitual smokers of marijuana, cocaine, and/or tobacco. Journal of the National Cancer Institute. 1998;**90**(16):1198-1205

[111] Fligiel SE, Roth MD, Kleerup EC, Barsky SH, Simmons MS, Tashkin DP. Tracheobronchial histopathology in habitual smokers of cocaine, marijuana, and/or tobacco. Chest. 1997;**112**(2):319-326

[112] Gong H Jr, Fligiel S, Tashkin DP, Barbers RG. Tracheobronchial changes in habitual, heavy smokers of marijuana with and without tobacco. The American review of respiratory disease. 1987;**136**(1):142-149

[113] Aldington S, Harwood M, Cox B, Weatherall M, Beckert L, Hansell A, et al. Cannabis use and risk of lung cancer: A case-control study. The European Respiratory Journal. 2008;**31**(2):280-286

[114] Callaghan RC, Allecbeck P, Sidorchuk A. Marijuana use and risk of lung cancer: A 40-year cohort study. Cancer Causes & Control. 2013;**24**:1811-1820

[115] Han B, Gfroerer JC, Colliver JD. Associations between duration of illicit drug use and health conditions: Results from the 2005-2007 national surveys on drug use and health. Annals of Epidemiology. 2010;**20**(4):289-297

[116] Hashibe M, Morgenstern H, Cui Y, Tashkin DP, Zhang ZF, Cozen W, et al. Marijuana use and the risk of lung and upper aerodigestive tract cancers: Results of a population-based case-control study. Cancer Epidemiology, Biomarkers & Prevention. 2006;**15**(10):1829-1834

[117] Sidney S Jr, CPQ, Friedman GD, Tekawa IS. Marijuana use and cancer incidence (California, United States). Cancer Causes & Control. 1997;**8**(5):722-728

[118] Zhang LR, Morgenstern H, Greenland S, Chang SC, Lazarus P, Teare MD, et al. Cannabis smoking and lung cancer risk: Pooled analysis in the International Lung Cancer Consortium. International Journal of Cancer. 2014;**136**(4):894-903

[119] Gieringer D. Waterpipe study. Multidisciplinary Assocation for Psycheldelic Studies (MAPS). 1996;**6**(3). https://maps.org/news-letters/v06n3/06359mj1.html

[120] Gieringer D, St. Laurent J, Goodrich S. Cannabis vaporizer combines efficient delivery of THC with effective suppression of pyrolytic compounds. Journal of Cannabis Therapeutics. 2004;**4**(1):7-27

[121] Lee ML, Novotny M, Bartle KD. Gas chromatography/mass spectrometric and nuclear magnetic resonance spectrometric studies of carcinogenic polynuclear aromatic hydrocarbons in tobacco and marijuana smoke condensates. Analytical Chemistry. 1976;**48**(2):405-416

[122] Sparacino CM, Hyldburg PA, Hughes TJ. Chemical and biological analysis of marijuana smoke condensate. NIDA Res Monogr. 1990;**99**:121-140.

[123] Callaghan RC, Allebeck P, Akre O, McGlynn KA, Sidorchuk A. Cannabis use and incidence of testicular cancer: A 42-year follow-up of Swedish men between 1970 and 2011. Cancer

Epidemiology, Biomarkers & Prevention. 2017;**26**(11):1644-1652

[124] Daling JR, Doody DR, Sun X, Trabert BL, Weiss NS, Chen C, et al. Association of marijuana use and the incidence of testicular germ cell tumors. Cancer. 2009;**115**(6):1215-1223

[125] Gurney J, Shaw C, Stanley J, Signal V, Sarfati D. Cannabis exposure and risk of testicular cancer: A systematic review and meta-analysis. BMC Cancer. 2015;**15**:897

[126] Lacson JCA, Carroll JD, Tuazon E, Castelao EJ, Bernstein L, Cortessis VK. Population-based case-control study of recreational drug use and testis cancer risk confirms an association between marijuana use and nonseminoma risk. Cancer. 2012;**118**(21):5374-5383

[127] Trabert B, Sigurdson AJ, Sweeney AM, Strom SS, McGlynn KA. Marijuana use and testicular germ cell tumors. Cancer. 2011;**117**(4):848-853

[128] Barber PA, Pridmore HM, Krishnamurthy V, Roberts S, Spriggs DA, Carter KN, et al. Cannabis, ischemic stroke, and transient ischemic attack: A case-control study. Stroke. 2013;**44**(8):2327-2329

[129] Desai R, Singh S, Patel K, Goyal H, Shah M, Mansuri Z, et al. Stroke in young cannabis users (18-49 years): National trends in hospitalizations and outcomes. International Journal of Stroke. 2020;**15**(5):535-539

[130] Dutta T, Ryan KA, Thompson O, Lopez H, Fecteau N, Sparks MJ, et al. Marijuana use and the risk of early ischemic stroke: The stroke prevention in young adults study. Stroke. 2021;**52**(10):3184-3190

[131] Falkstedt D, Wolff V, Allebeck P, Hemmingsson T, Danielsson AK. Cannabis, tobacco, alcohol use, and the risk of early stroke: A population-based Cohort Study of 45 000 Swedish men. Stroke. 2017;**48**(2):265-270

[132] Geller T, Loftis L, Brink DS. Cerebellar infarction in adolescent males associated with acute marijuana use. Pediatrics. 2004;**113**(4):e365-e370

[133] Hackam DG. Cannabis and stroke: Systematic appraisal of case reports. Stroke. 2015;**46**(3):852-856

[134] Hemachandra D, McKetin R, Cherbuin N, Anstey KJ. Heavy cannabis users at elevated risk of stroke: Evidence from a general population survey. Australian and New Zealand Journal of Public Health. 2016;**40**(3):226-230

[135] Kalla A, Krishnamoorthy PM, Gopalakrishnan A, Figueredo VM. Cannabis use predicts risks of heart failure and cerebrovascular accidents: Results from the National Inpatient Sample. Journal of Cardiovascular Medicine (Hagerstown, Md.). 2018;**19**(9):480-484

[136] Reis JP, Auer R, Bancks MP, Goff DC Jr, Lewis CE, Pletcher MJ, et al. Cumulative lifetime marijuana use and incident cardiovascular disease in middle age: The coronary artery risk development in young adults (CARDIA) study. American Journal of Public Health. 2017;**107**(4):601-606

[137] Rumalla K, Reddy AY, Mittal MK. Recreational marijuana use and acute ischemic stroke: A population-based analysis of hospitalized patients in the United States. Journal of the Neurological Sciences. 2016;**364**:191-196

[138] Shah S, Patel S, Paulraj S, Chaudhuri D. Association of marijuana use and cardiovascular disease: A behavioral risk factor surveillance system data analysis of 133,706 US adults.

The American Journal of Medicine. 2020;**134**(5):614-620

[139] Thanvi BR, Treadwell SD. Cannabis and stroke: Is there a link? Postgraduate Medical Journal. 2009;**85**(1000):80-83

[140] Vin-Raviv N, Akinyemiju T, Meng Q, Sakhuja S, Hayward R. Marijuana use and inpatient outcomes among hospitalized patients: Analysis of the nationwide inpatient sample database. Cancer Medicine. 2017;**6**(1):320-329

[141] Westover AN, McBride S, Haley RW. Stroke in young adults who abuse amphetamines or cocaine: A population-based study of hospitalized patients. Archives of General Psychiatry. 2007;**64**(4):495-502

[142] Wolff V, Armspach J-P, Lauer V, Rouyer O, Bataillard M, Marescaux C, et al. Cannabis-related stroke: Myth or reality? Stroke; A Journal of Cerebral Circulation. 2013;**44**(2):558-563

[143] Yang PK, Odom EC, Patel R, Loustalot F, Coleman King S. Nonmedical marijuana use and cardiovascular events: A systematic review. Public Health Reports. 2021;**137**(1):62-71. DOI: 10.1177/0033354920988285

[144] Parekh T, Pemmasani S, Desai R. Marijuana use among young adults (18-44 years of age) and risk of stroke: A behavioral risk factor surveillance system survey analysis. Stroke. 2020;**51**(1):308-310

[145] van Winkel R, Genetic R. Outcome of Psychosis I. Family-based analysis of genetic variation underlying psychosis-inducing effects of cannabis: Sibling analysis and proband follow-up. Archives of General Psychiatry. 2011;**68**(2):148-157

[146] Bosker WM, Kuypers KP, Theunissen EL, Surinx A, Blankespoor RJ, Skopp G, et al. Medicinal Delta(9) -tetrahydrocannabinol (dronabinol) impairs on-the-road driving performance of occasional and heavy cannabis users but is not detected in Standard Field Sobriety Tests. Addiction. 2012;**107**(10):1837-1844

[147] Curran HV, Brignell C, Fletcher S, Middleton P, Henry J. Cognitive and subjective dose-response effects of acute oral Delta 9-tetrahydrocannabinol (THC) in infrequent cannabis users. Psychopharmacology. 2002;**164**(1):61-70

[148] Lile JA, Kelly TH, Charnigo RJ, Stinchcomb AL, Hays LR. Pharmacokinetic and pharmacodynamic profile of supratherapeutic oral doses of Delta(9) -THC in cannabis users. Journal of Clinical Pharmacology. 2013;**53**(7):680-690

[149] Newmeyer MN, Swortwood MJ, Barnes AJ, Abulseoud OA, Scheidweiler KB, Huestis MA. Free and glucuronide whole blood cannabinoids' pharmacokinetics after controlled smoked, vaporized, and oral cannabis administration in frequent and occasional cannabis users: Identification of recent cannabis intake. Clinical Chemistry. 2016;**62**(12):1579-1592

[150] Newmeyer MN, Swortwood MJ, Andersson M, Abulseoud OA, Scheidweiler KB, Huestis MA. Cannabis edibles: Blood and oral fluid cannabinoid pharmacokinetics and evaluation of oral fluid screening devices for predicting delta(9)-tetrahydrocannabinol in blood and oral fluid following cannabis brownie administration. Clinical Chemistry. 2017;**63**(3):647-662

[151] Vandrey R, Herrmann ES, Mitchell JM, Bigelow GE, Flegel R, LoDico C, et al. Pharmacokinetic profile of oral cannabis in humans: Blood and oral fluid disposition and relation to

pharmacodynamic outcomes. Journal of Analytical Toxicology. 2017;**41**(2):83-99

[152] Bidwell LC, Karoly HC, Torres MO, Master A, Bryan AD, Hutchison KE. A naturalistic study of orally administered vs. inhaled legal market cannabis: Cannabinoids exposure, intoxication, and impairment. Psychopharmacology. 2021;**239**(2):385-397

[153] Menetrey A, Augsburger M, Favrat B, Pin MA, Rothuizen LE, Appenzeller M, et al. Assessment of driving capability through the use of clinical and psychomotor tests in relation to blood cannabinoids levels following oral administration of 20 mg dronabinol or of a cannabis decoction made with 20 or 60 mg Delta9-THC. Journal of Analytical Toxicology. 2005;**29**(5):327-338

[154] Schlienz NJ, Spindle TR, Cone EJ, Herrmann ES, Bigelow GE, Mitchell JM, et al. Pharmacodynamic dose effects of oral cannabis ingestion in healthy adults who infrequently use cannabis. Drug and Alcohol Dependence. 2020;**211**:107969

[155] Berghaus G, Sticht G, Grellner W. Meta-analysis of Empirical Studies Concerning the Effects of Medicines and Illegal Drugs Including Pharmacokinetics on Safe Driving. Center for Traffic Sciences at the University of Wurzburg; Federal Highway Research Institute. 2011

[156] Huestis MA, Henningfield JE, Cone EJ. Blood cannabinoids. I. Absorption of THC and formation of 11-OH-THC and THCCOOH during and after smoking marijuana. Journal of Analytical Toxicology. 1992;**16**(5):276-282

[157] Ramaekers JG, Moeller MR, van Ruitenbeek P, Theunissen EL, Schneider E, Kauert G. Cognition and motor control as a function of Delta9-THC concentration in serum and oral fluid: Limits of impairment. Drug and Alcohol Dependence. 2006;**85**(2):114-122

[158] Reeve VC, Grant JD, Robertson W, Gillespie HK, Hollister LE. Plasma concentrations of delta-9-tetrahydrocannabinol and impaired motor function. Drug and Alcohol Dependence. 1983;**11**(2):167-175

[159] Spindle TR, Cone EJ, Schlienz NJ, Mitchell JM, Bigelow GE, Flegel R, et al. Acute pharmacokinetic profile of smoked and vaporized cannabis in human blood and oral fluid. Journal of Analytical Toxicology. 2019;**43**(4):233-258

[160] Abrams DI, Vizoso HP, Shade SB, Jay C, Kelly ME, Benowitz NL. Vaporization as a smokeless cannabis delivery system: A pilot study. Clinical Pharmacology and Therapeutics. 2007;**82**(5):572-578

[161] Cone EJ, Bigelow GE, Herrmann ES, Mitchell JM, LoDico C, Flegel R, et al. Nonsmoker exposure to secondhand cannabis smoke. III. Oral fluid and blood drug concentrations and corresponding subjective effects. Journal of Analytical Toxicology. 2015;**39**(7):497-509

[162] Herrmann ES, Cone EJ, Mitchell JM, Bigelow GE, LoDico C, Flegel R, et al. Non-smoker exposure to secondhand cannabis smoke II: Effect of room ventilation on the physiological, subjective, and behavioral/cognitive effects. Drug and Alcohol Dependence. 2015;**151**:194-202

[163] Law B, Mason PA, Moffat AC, King LJ, Marks V. Passive inhalation of cannabis smoke. The Journal of Pharmacy and Pharmacology. 1984;**36**(9):578-581

[164] Mason AP, Perez-Reyes M, McBay AJ, Foltz RL. Cannabinoids in plasma after passive inhalation of marijuana smoke.

Journal of the American Medical Association. 1983;**249**(4):475-476

[165] Mule SJ, Lomax P, Gross SJ. Active and realistic passive marijuana exposure tested by three immunoassays and GC/MS in urine. Journal of Analytical Toxicology. 1988;**12**(3):113-116

[166] Niedbala RS, Kardos KW, Fritch DF, Kunsman KP, Blum KA, Newland GA, et al. Passive cannabis smoke exposure and oral fluid testing. II. Two studies of extreme cannabis smoke exposure in a motor vehicle. Journal of Analytical Toxicology. 2005;**29**(7):607-615

[167] Niedbala S, Kardos K, Salamone S, Fritch D, Bronsgeest M, Cone EJ. Passive cannabis smoke exposure and oral fluid testing. Journal of Analytical Toxicology. 2004;**28**(7):546-552

[168] Perez-Reyes M, di Guiseppi S, Davis KH. Passive inhalation of marijuana smoke and urinary excretion cannabinoids. Journal of the American Medical Association. 1983;**249**(4):475

[169] Rohrich J, Schimmel I, Zorntlein S, Becker J, Drobnik S, Kaufmann T, et al. Concentrations of delta9-tetrahydrocannabinol and 11-nor-9-carboxytetrahydrocannabinol in blood and urine after passive exposure to Cannabis smoke in a coffee shop. Journal of Analytical Toxicology. 2010;**34**(4):196-203

[170] Chihuri S, Li G. Direct and indirect effects of marijuana use on the risk of fatal 2-vehicle crash initiation. Injury Epidemiology. 2020;**7**(1):49

[171] Chihuri S, Li G, Chen Q. Interaction of marijuana and alcohol on fatal motor vehicle crash risk: A case-control study. Injury Epidemiology. 2017;**4**(1):8

[172] Li G, Chihuri S, Brady JE. Role of alcohol and marijuana use in the initiation of fatal two-vehicle crashes. Annals of Epidemiology. 2017;**27**(5):342-7.e1

[173] Drummer OH, Gerostamoulos J, Batziris H, Chu M, Caplehorn J, Robertson MD, et al. The involvement of drugs in drivers of motor vehicles killed in Australian road traffic crashes. Accident Analysis & Prevention. 2004;**36**(2):239-248

[174] Drummer OH, Gerostamoulos D, Di Rago M, Woodford NW, Morris C, Frederiksen T, et al. Odds of culpability associated with use of impairing drugs in injured drivers in Victoria, Australia. Accident Analysis & Prevention. 2020;**135**:105389

[175] Dubois S, Mullen N, Weaver B, Bedard M. The combined effects of alcohol and cannabis on driving: Impact on crash risk. Forensic Science International. 2015;**248**:94-100

[176] Fierro I, González-Luque JC, Álvarez FJ. The relationship between observed signs of impairment and THC concentration in oral fluid. Drug and Alcohol Dependence. 2014;**144**:231-238

[177] Hartman RL, Brown TL, Milavetz G, Spurgin A, Pierce RS, Gorelick DA, et al. Cannabis effects on driving lateral control with and without alcohol. Drug and Alcohol Dependence. 2015;**154**:25-37

[178] Laumon B, Gadegbeku B, Martin JL, Biecheler MB, Group SAM. Cannabis intoxication and fatal road crashes in France: Population based case-control study. BMJ. 2005;**331**(7529):1371

[179] Mura P, Kintz P, Ludes B, Gaulier JM, Marquet P, Martin-Dupont S, et al. Comparison of the prevalence of alcohol, cannabis and other drugs between 900 injured drivers and 900 control subjects: Results of a French

collaborative study. Forensic Science International. 2003;**133**(1-2):79-85

[180] Poulsen H, Moar R, Pirie R. The culpability of drivers killed in New Zealand road crashes and their use of alcohol and other drugs. Accident; Analysis and Prevention. 2014;**67**:119-128

[181] Sewell RA, Poling J, Sofuoglu M. The effect of cannabis compared with alcohol on driving. The American Journal on Addictions. 2009;**18**(3):185-193

[182] Asbridge M, Hayden JA, Cartwright JL. Acute cannabis consumption and motor vehicle collision risk: Systematic review of observational studies and meta-analysis. BMJ. 2012;**344**:e536

[183] Del Balzo G, Gottardo R, Mengozzi S, Dorizzi RM, Bortolotti F, Appolonova S, et al. "Positive" urine testing for Cannabis is associated with increased risk of traffic crashes. Journal of Pharmaceutical and Biomedical Analysis. 2018;**151**:71-74

[184] Gjerde H, Strand MC, Morland J. Driving under the influence of non-alcohol drugs—An update part I: Epidemiological studies. Forensic Science Review. 2015;**27**(2):89-113

[185] Hartman RL, Huestis MA. Cannabis effects on driving skills. Clinical Chemistry. 2013;**59**(3):478-492

[186] Lowenstein SR, Koziol-McLain J. Drugs and traffic crash responsibility: A study of injured motorists in Colorado. The Journal of Trauma: Injury, Infection, and Critical Care. 2001;**50**(2):313-320

[187] Preuss UW, Huestis MA, Schneider M, Hermann D, Lutz B, Hasan A, et al. Cannabis use and car crashes: A review. Frontiers in Psychiatry. 2021;**12**:643315

[188] Rogeberg O, Elvik R. The effects of cannabis intoxication on motor vehicle collision revisited and revised. Addiction. 2016;**111**(8):1348-1359

[189] Kuypers KP, Legrand SA, Ramaekers JG, Verstraete AG. A case-control study estimating accident risk for alcohol, medicines and illegal drugs. PLoS One. 2012;**7**(8):e43496

[190] Berghaus G, Scheer N, Schmidt P. Effects of cannabis on psychomotor skills and driving performance—a metaanalysis of experimental studies. 1995. Available from: http://casr.adelaide.edu.au/T95/paper/s16p2.html

[191] Hart CL, van Gorp W, Haney M, Foltin RW, Fischman MW. Effects of acute smoked marijuana on complex cognitive performance. Neuropsychopharmacology. 2001;**25**(5):757-765

[192] Hunault CC, Mensinga TT, Bocker KB, Schipper CM, Kruidenier M, Leenders ME, et al. Cognitive and psychomotor effects in males after smoking a combination of tobacco and cannabis containing up to 69 mg delta-9-tetrahydrocannabinol (THC). Psychopharmacology. 2009;**204**(1):85-94

[193] Kelly TH, Foltin RW, Emurian CS, Fischman MW. Performance-based testing for drugs of abuse: Dose and time profiles of marijuana, amphetamine, alcohol, and diazepam. Journal of Analytical Toxicology. 1993;**17**(5):264-272

[194] Lenne MG, Dietze PM, Triggs TJ, Walmsley S, Murphy B, Redman JR. The effects of cannabis and alcohol on simulated arterial driving: Influences of driving experience and task demand. Accident; Analysis and Prevention. 2010;**42**(3):859-866

[195] Micallef J, Dupouey J, Jouve E, Truillet R, Lacarelle B, Taillard J, et al. Cannabis smoking impairs driving performance on the simulator and real driving: A randomized, double-blind, placebo-controlled, crossover trial. Fundamental & Clinical Pharmacology. 2018;**32**(5):558-570

[196] Ramaekers JG, Kauert G, Theunissen EL, Toennes SW, Moeller MR. Neurocognitive performance during acute THC intoxication in heavy and occasional cannabis users. Journal of Psychopharmacology. 2009;**23**(3):266-277

[197] Ramaekers JG, Kauert G, van Ruitenbeek P, Theunissen EL, Schneider E, Moeller MR. High-potency marijuana impairs executive function and inhibitory motor control. Neuropsychopharmacology. 2006;**31**(10):2296-2303

[198] Ronen A, Chassidim HS, Gershon P, Parmet Y, Rabinovich A, Bar-Hamburger R, et al. The effect of alcohol, THC and their combination on perceived effects, willingness to drive and performance of driving and non-driving tasks. Accident; Analysis and Prevention. 2010;**42**(6):1855-1865

[199] Schwope DM, Bosker WM, Ramaekers JG, Gorelick DA, Huestis MA. Psychomotor performance, subjective and physiological effects and whole blood Delta(9)-tetrahydrocannabinol concentrations in heavy, chronic cannabis smokers following acute smoked cannabis. Journal of Analytical Toxicology. 2012;**36**(6):405-412

[200] Weinstein A, Brickner O, Lerman H, Greemland M, Bloch M, Lester H, et al. A study investigating the acute dose-response effects of 13 mg and 17 mg Delta 9-tetrahydrocannabinol on cognitive-motor skills, subjective and autonomic measures in regular users of marijuana. Journal of Psychopharmacology. 2008;**22**(4):441-451

[201] Vindenes V, Strand DH, Kristoffersen L, Boix F, Morland J. Has the intake of THC by cannabis users changed over the last decade? Evidence of increased exposure by analysis of blood THC concentrations in impaired drivers. Forensic Science International. 2013;**226**(1-3):197-201

[202] Arkell TR, Vinckenbosch F, Kevin RC, Theunissen EL, McGregor IS, Ramaekers JG. Effect of cannabidiol and Δ9-tetrahydrocannabinol on driving performance: A randomized clinical trial. Journal of the American Medical Association. 2020;**324**(21):2177-2186

[203] Brooks-Russell A, Brown T, Friedman K, Wrobel J, Schwarz J, Dooley G, et al. Simulated driving performance among daily and occasional cannabis users. Accident; Analysis and Prevention. 2021;**160**:106326

[204] Grotenhermen F, Leson G, Berghaus G, Drummer OH, Kruger HP, Longo M, et al. Developing limits for driving under cannabis. Addiction. 2007;**102**(12):1910-1917

[205] Brubacher JR, Chan H, Erdelyi S, Macdonald S, Asbridge M, Mann RE, et al. Cannabis use as a risk factor for causing motor vehicle crashes: a prospective study. Addiction. 2019;**114**(9):1616-1626

[206] Ortiz-Peregrina S, Ortiz C, Castro-Torres JJ, Jiménez JR, Anera RG. Effects of smoking cannabis on visual function and driving performance. A driving-simulator based study. International Journal of Environmental Research and Public Health. 2020;**17**(23):9033

[207] Tank A, Tietz T, Daldrup T, Schwender H, Hellen F, Ritz-Timme S, et al. On the impact of cannabis consumption on traffic safety: A driving simulator study with habitual cannabis consumers. International Journal of Legal Medicine. 2019;**133**(5):1411-1420

[208] Huestis MA. Human cannabinoid pharmacokinetics. Chemistry & Biodiversity. 2007;**4**(8):1770-1804

[209] Allen JH, de Moore GM, Heddle R, Twartz JC. Cannabinoid hyperemesis: Cyclical hyperemesis in association with chronic cannabis abuse. Gut. 2004;**53**(11):1566-1570

[210] Contreras Narvaez C, Mola Gilbert M, Batlle de Santiago E, Bigas Farreres J, Gine Serven E, Canete CJ. Cannabinoid hyperemesis syndrome. A report of six new cases and a summary of previous reports. Adicciones. 2016;**28**(2):90-98

[211] Kim HS, Anderson JD, Saghafi O, Heard KJ, Monte AA. Cyclic vomiting presentations following marijuana liberalization in Colorado. Academic Emergency Medicine. 2015;**22**(6):694-699

[212] Lonsdale H, Kimsey KM, Brown JM, Dey A, Peck J, Son S, et al. Pediatric cannabinoid hyperemesis: A single institution 10-year case series. The Journal of Adolescent Health. 2021;**68**(2):255-261

[213] Monte AA, Shelton SK, Mills E, Saben J, Hopkinson A, Sonn B, et al. Acute illness associated with cannabis use, by route of exposure: An observational study. Annals of Internal Medicine. 2019;**170**(8):531-537

[214] Rotella JA, Ferretti OG, Raisi E, Seet HR, Sarkar S. Cannabinoid hyperemesis syndrome: A 6-year audit of adult presentations to an urban district hospital. Emergency Medicine Australasia. 2022;**34**(4):578-583

[215] Simonetto DA, Oxentenko AS, Herman ML, Szostek JH. Cannabinoid hyperemesis: A case series of 98 patients. Mayo Clinic Proceedings. 2012;**87**(2):114-119

[216] Soriano-Co M, Batke M, Cappell MS. The cannabis hyperemesis syndrome characterized by persistent nausea and vomiting, abdominal pain, and compulsive bathing associated with chronic marijuana use: A report of eight cases in the United States. Digestive Diseases and Sciences. 2010;**55**(11):3113-3119

[217] von Both I, Santos B. Death of a young woman with cyclic vomiting: A case report. Forensic Science, Medicine, and Pathology. 2021;**17**(4):715-722

[218] Wallace EA, Andrews SE, Garmany CL, Jelley MJ. Cannabinoid hyperemesis syndrome: Literature review and proposed diagnosis and treatment algorithm. Southern Medical Journal. 2011;**104**(9):659-664

[219] Donnino MW, Cocchi MN, Miller J, Fisher J. Cannabinoid hyperemesis: A case series. The Journal of Emergency Medicine. 2011;**40**(4):e63-e66

[220] Venkatesan T, Levinthal DJ, Li BUK, Tarbell SE, Adams KA, Issenman RM, et al. Role of chronic cannabis use: Cyclic vomiting syndrome vs cannabinoid hyperemesis syndrome. Neurogastroenterology & Motility. 2019;**31**(Suppl 2):e13606

[221] Epstein-Ngo QM, Cunningham RM, Whiteside LK, Chermack ST, Booth BM, Zimmerman MA, et al. A daily calendar analysis of substance use and dating

violence among high risk urban youth. Drug and Alcohol Dependence. 2013;**130**(1-3):194-200

[222] Nabors EL. Drug use and intimate partner violence among college students: An in-depth exploration. Journal of Interpersonal Violence. 2010;**25**(6):1043-1063

[223] Rothman EF, Johnson RM, Azrael D, Hall DM, Weinberg J. Perpetration of physical assault against dating partners, peers, and siblings among a locally representative sample of high school students in Boston, Massachusetts. Archives of Pediatrics & Adolescent Medicine. 2010;**164**(12):1118-1124

[224] Shorey RC, Stuart GL, Moore TM, McNulty JK. The temporal relationship between alcohol, marijuana, angry affect, and dating violence perpetration: A daily diary study with female college students. Psychology of Addictive Behaviors. 2014;**28**(2):516-523

[225] Testa M, Hoffman JH, Leonard KE. Female intimate partner violence perpetration: Stability and predictors of mutual and nonmutual aggression across the first year of college. Aggressive Behavior. 2011;**37**(4):362-373

[226] Testa M, Derrick JL, Wang W, Leonard KE, Kubiak A, Brown WC, et al. Does marijuana contribute to intimate partner aggression? Temporal effects in a community sample of marijuana-using couples. Journal of Studies on Alcohol and Drugs. 2018;**79**(3):432-440

[227] Auer R, Vittinghoff E, Yaffe K, Kunzi A, Kertesz SG, Levine DA, et al. Association between lifetime marijuana use and cognitive function in middle age: The coronary artery risk development in young adults (CARDIA) study. JAMA Internal Medicine. 2016;**176**(3):352-361

[228] Pope HG Jr, Gruber AJ, Hudson JI, Huestis MA, Yurgelun-Todd D. Neuropsychological performance in long-term cannabis users. Archives of General Psychiatry. 2001;**58**(10):909-915

[229] Rodgers J, Buchanan T, Scholey AB, Heffernan TM, Ling J, Parrott A. Differential effects of Ecstasy and cannabis on self-reports of memory ability: A web-based study. Human Psychopharmacology. 2001;**16**(8):619-625

[230] Roebke PV, Vadhan NP, Brooks DJ, Levin FR. Verbal learning in marijuana users seeking treatment: A comparison between depressed and non-depressed samples. The American Journal of Drug and Alcohol Abuse. 2014;**40**(4):274-279

[231] Sanchez-Torres AM, Basterra V, Rosa A, Fananas L, Zarzuela A, Ibanez B, et al. Lifetime cannabis use and cognition in patients with schizophrenia spectrum disorders and their unaffected siblings. European Archives of Psychiatry and Clinical Neuroscience. 2013;**263**(8):643-653

[232] Schoeler T, Kambeitz J, Behlke I, Murray R, Bhattacharyya S. The effects of cannabis on memory function in users with and without a psychotic disorder: Findings from a combined meta-analysis. Psychological Medicine. 2016;**46**(1):177-188

[233] Solowij N. Cognitive functioning of long-term heavy cannabis users seeking treatment. Journal of the American Medical Association. 2002;**287**(9):1123

[234] Tamm L, Epstein JN, Lisdahl KM, Molina B, Tapert S, Hinshaw SP, et al. Impact of ADHD and cannabis use on executive functioning in young adults. Drug and Alcohol Dependence. 2013;**133**(2):607-614

[235] Thames AD, Arbid N, Sayegh P. Cannabis use and neurocognitive functioning in a non-clinical sample of users. Addictive Behaviors. 2014;**39**(5):994-999

[236] Curran HV, Hindocha C, Morgan CJA, Shaban N, Das RK, Freeman TP. Which biological and self-report measures of cannabis use predict cannabis dependency and acute psychotic-like effects? Psychological Medicine. 2019;**49**(9):1574-1580

[237] D'Souza DC, Perry E, MacDougall L, Ammerman Y, Cooper T, Wu YT, et al. The psychotomimetic effects of intravenous delta-9-tetrahydrocannabinol in healthy individuals: Implications for psychosis. Neuropsychopharmacology. 2004;**29**(8):1558-1572

[238] Englund A, Atakan Z, Kralj A, Tunstall N, Murray R, Morrison P. The effect of five day dosing with THCV on THC-induced cognitive, psychological and physiological effects in healthy male human volunteers: A placebo-controlled, double-blind, crossover pilot trial. Journal of Psychopharmacology. 2016;**30**(2):140-151

[239] Mason O, Morgan CJ, Dhiman SK, Patel A, Parti N, Patel A, et al. Acute cannabis use causes increased psychotomimetic experiences in individuals prone to psychosis. Psychological Medicine. 2009;**39**(6):951-956

[240] Morrison PD, Zois V, McKeown DA, Lee TD, Holt DW, Powell JF, et al. The acute effects of synthetic intravenous Delta9-tetrahydrocannabinol on psychosis, mood and cognitive functioning. Psychological Medicine. 2009;**39**(10):1607-1616

[241] Nestoros JN, Vakonaki E, Tzatzarakis MN, Alegakis A, Skondras MD, Tsatsakis AM. Long lasting effects of chronic heavy cannabis abuse. The American Journal on Addictions. 2017;**26**(4):335-342

[242] Morrison PD, Stone JM. Synthetic delta-9-tetrahydrocannabinol elicits schizophrenia-like negative symptoms which are distinct from sedation. Human Psychopharmacology. 2011;**26**(1):77-80

[243] Morgan CJ, Rothwell E, Atkinson H, Mason O, Curran HV. Hyper-priming in cannabis users: A naturalistic study of the effects of cannabis on semantic memory function. Psychiatry Research. 2010;**176**(2-3):213-218

[244] Giordano GN, Ohlsson H, Sundquist K, Sundquist J, Kendler KS. The association between cannabis abuse and subsequent schizophrenia: A Swedish national co-relative control study. Psychological Medicine. 2015;**45**(2):407-414

[245] Hjorthøj C, Posselt CM, Nordentoft M. Development over time of the population-attributable risk fraction for cannabis use disorder in schizophrenia in Denmark. JAMA Psychiatry. 2021;**78**(9):1013-1019

[246] Nielsen SM, Toftdahl NG, Nordentoft M, Hjorthoj C. Association between alcohol, cannabis, and other illicit substance abuse and risk of developing schizophrenia: A nationwide population based register study. Psychological Medicine. 2017;**47**(9):1668-1677

[247] Sideli L, Fisher HL, Murray RM, Sallis H, Russo M, Stilo SA, et al. Interaction between cannabis consumption and childhood abuse in psychotic disorders: Preliminary findings on the role of different patterns of cannabis use. Early Intervention in Psychiatry. 2018;**12**(2):135-142

[248] Blanco C, Hasin DS, Wall MM, Florez-Salamanca L, Hoertel N, Wang S, et al. Cannabis use and risk of psychiatric disorders: prospective evidence from a US national longitudinal study. JAMA Psychiatry. 2016;**73**(4):388-395

[249] Buu A, Hu YH, Pampati S, Arterberry BJ, Lin HC. Predictive validity of cannabis consumption measures: Results from a national longitudinal study. Addictive Behaviors. 2017;**73**:36-40

[250] Callaghan RC, Sanches M, Kish SJ. Quantity and frequency of cannabis use in relation to cannabis-use disorder and cannabis-related problems. Drug and Alcohol Dependence. 2020;**217**:108271

[251] Leung J, Chan GCK, Hides L, Hall WD. What is the prevalence and risk of cannabis use disorders among people who use cannabis? A systematic review and meta-analysis. Addictive Behaviors. 2020;**109**:106479

[252] Lopez-Quintero C, Perez de los Cobos J, Hasin DS, Okuda M, Wang S, Grant BF, et al. Probability and predictors of transition from first use to dependence on nicotine, alcohol, cannabis, and cocaine: Results of the National Epidemiologic Survey on Alcohol and Related Conditions (NESARC). Drug and Alcohol Dependence. 2011;**115**(1-2):120-130

[253] Buckner JD, Zvolensky MJ, Ecker AH, Schmidt NB, Lewis EM, Paulus DJ, et al. Integrated cognitive behavioral therapy for comorbid cannabis use and anxiety disorders: A pilot randomized controlled trial. Behaviour Research and Therapy. 2019;**115**:38-45

[254] Budney AJ, Higgins ST, Radonovich KJ, Novy PL. Adding voucher-based incentives to coping skills and motivational enhancement improves outcomes during treatment for marijuana dependence. Journal of Consulting and Clinical Psychology. 2000;**68**(6):1051-1061

[255] Budney AJ, Stanger C, Tilford JM, Scherer EB, Brown PC, Li Z, et al. Computer-assisted behavioral therapy and contingency management for cannabis use disorder. Psychology of Addictive Behaviors. 2015;**29**(3):501-511

[256] Copeland J, Swift W, Roffman R, Stephens R. A randomized controlled trial of brief cognitive-behavioral interventions for cannabis use disorder. Journal of Substance Abuse Treatment. 2001;**21**(2):55-64; discussion 5-6

[257] Rooke S, Copeland J, Norberg M, Hine D, McCambridge J. Effectiveness of a self-guided web-based cannabis treatment program: Randomized controlled trial. Journal of Medical Internet Research. 2013;**15**(2):e26

[258] Budney AJ, Moore BA, Vandrey RG, Hughes JR. The time course and significance of cannabis withdrawal. Journal of Abnormal Psychology. 2003;**112**(3):393-402

[259] Budney AJ, Novy PL, Hughes JR. Marijuana withdrawal among adults seeking treatment for marijuana dependence. Addiction. 1999;**94**(9):1311-1322

[260] Budney AJ, Radonovich KJ, Higgins ST, Wong CJ. Adults seeking treatment for marijuana dependence: A comparison with cocaine-dependent treatment seekers. Experimental and Clinical Psychopharmacology. 1998;**6**(4):419-426

[261] Budney AJ, Vandrey RG, Hughes JR, Moore BA, Bahrenburg B. Oral delta-9-tetrahydrocannabinol suppresses cannabis withdrawal symptoms.

Drug and Alcohol Dependence. 2007;**86**(1):22-29

[262] Budney AJ, Vandrey RG, Hughes JR, Thostenson JD, Bursac Z. Comparison of cannabis and tobacco withdrawal: Severity and contribution to relapse. Journal of Substance Abuse Treatment. 2008;**35**(4):362-368

[263] Cousijn J, van Duijvenvoorde ACK. Cognitive and mental health predictors of withdrawal severity during an active attempt to cut down cannabis use. Frontiers in Psychiatry. 2018;**9**:301

[264] Greene MC, Kelly JF. The prevalence of cannabis withdrawal and its influence on adolescents' treatment response and outcomes: a 12-month prospective investigation. Journal of Addiction Medicine. 2014;**8**(5):359-367

[265] Hasin DS, Keyes KM, Alderson D, Wang S, Aharonovich E, Grant BF. Cannabis withdrawal in the United States: Results from NESARC. The Journal of Clinical Psychiatry. 2008;**69**(9):1354-1363

[266] Herrmann ES, Weerts EM, Vandrey R. Sex differences in cannabis withdrawal symptoms among treatment-seeking cannabis users. Experimental and Clinical Psychopharmacology. 2015;**23**(6):415-421

[267] Livne O, Shmulewitz D, Lev-Ran S, Hasin DS. DSM-5 cannabis withdrawal syndrome: Demographic and clinical correlates in U.S. adults. Drug and Alcohol Dependence. 2019;**195**:170-177

[268] Vandrey R, Budney AJ, Kamon JL, Stanger C. Cannabis withdrawal in adolescent treatment seekers. Drug and Alcohol Dependence. 2005;**78**(2):205-210

[269] Vandrey RG, Budney AJ, Hughes JR, Liguori A. A within-subject comparison of withdrawal symptoms during abstinence from cannabis, tobacco, and both substances. Drug and Alcohol Dependence. 2008;**92**(1-3):48-54

[270] Vandrey RG, Budney AJ, Moore BA, Hughes JR. A cross-study comparison of cannabis and tobacco withdrawal. The American Journal on Addictions. 2005;**14**(1):54-63

[271] Betts KS, Kisely S, Alati R. Prenatal cannabis use disorders and offspring primary and secondary educational outcomes. Addiction. 2022;**117**(2):425-432

[272] Fried PA, Watkinson B, Siegel LS. Reading and language in 9- to 12-year olds prenatally exposed to cigarettes and marijuana. Neurotoxicology and Teratology. 1997;**19**(3):171-183

[273] Goldschmidt L, Richardson GA, Cornelius MD, Day NL. Prenatal marijuana and alcohol exposure and academic achievement at age 10. Neurotoxicology and Teratology. 2004;**26**(4):521-532

[274] Goldschmidt L, Richardson GA, Willford JA, Severtson SG, Day NL. School achievement in 14-year-old youths prenatally exposed to marijuana. Neurotoxicology and Teratology. 2012;**34**(1):161-167

[275] Smith AM, Fried PA, Hogan MJ, Cameron I. Effects of prenatal marijuana on response inhibition: An fMRI study of young adults. Neurotoxicology and Teratology. 2004;**26**(4):533-542

[276] Amoretti S, Verdolini N, Varo C, Mezquida G, Sánchez-Torres AM, Vieta E, et al. Is the effect of cognitive reserve in longitudinal outcomes in first-episode psychoses dependent on the use of cannabis? Journal of Affective Disorders. 2022;**302**:83-93

[277] Torres CA, Medina-Kirchner C, O'Malley KY, Hart CL. Totality of the evidence suggests prenatal cannabis exposure does not lead to cognitive impairments: A systematic and critical review. Frontiers in Psychology. 2020;**11**:816

[278] Willford JA, Chandler LS, Goldschmidt L, Day NL. Effects of prenatal tobacco, alcohol and marijuana exposure on processing speed, visual-motor coordination, and interhemispheric transfer. Neurotoxicology and Teratology. 2010;**32**(6):580-588

[279] Day NL, Richardson GA, Goldschmidt L, Robles N, Taylor PM, Stoffer DS, et al. Effect of prenatal marijuana exposure on the cognitive development of offspring at age three. Neurotoxicology and Teratology. 1994;**16**(2):169-175

[280] Goldschmidt L, Richardson GA, Willford J, Day NL. Prenatal marijuana exposure and intelligence test performance at age 6. Journal of the American Academy of Child and Adolescent Psychiatry. 2008;**47**(3):254-263

[281] Eiden RD, Zhao J, Casey M, Shisler S, Schuetze P, Colder CR. Pre- and postnatal tobacco and cannabis exposure and child behavior problems: Bidirectional associations, joint effects, and sex differences. Drug and Alcohol Dependence. 2018;**185**:82-92

[282] El Marroun H, Tiemeier H, Steegers EA, Jaddoe VW, Hofman A, Verhulst FC, et al. Intrauterine cannabis exposure affects fetal growth trajectories: The Generation R Study. Journal of the American Academy of Child and Adolescent Psychiatry. 2009;**48**(12):1173-1181

[283] Fried PA, Smith AM. A literature review of the consequences of prenatal marihuana exposure. An emerging theme of a deficiency in aspects of executive function. Neurotoxicology and Teratology. 2001;**23**(1):1-11

[284] Noland JS, Singer LT, Short EJ, Minnes S, Arendt RE, Kirchner HL, et al. Prenatal drug exposure and selective attention in preschoolers. Neurotoxicology and Teratology. 2005;**27**(3):429-438

[285] Paul SE, Hatoum AS, Fine JD, Johnson EC, Hansen I, Karcher NR, et al. Associations between prenatal cannabis exposure and childhood outcomes: Results from the ABCD Study. JAMA Psychiatry. 2021;**78**(1):64-76

[286] Bandoli G, Jelliffe-Pawlowski L, Schumacher B, Baer RJ, Felder JN, Fuchs JD, et al. Cannabis-related diagnosis in pregnancy and adverse maternal and infant outcomes. Drug and Alcohol Dependence. 2021;**225**:108757

[287] Day N, Sambamoorthi U, Taylor P, Richardson G, Robles N, Jhon Y, et al. Prenatal marijuana use and neonatal outcome. Neurotoxicology and Teratology. 1991;**13**(3):329-334

[288] Forrester MB, Merz RD. Risk of selected birth defects with prenatal illicit drug use, Hawaii, 1986-2002. Journal of Toxicology and Environmental Health. Part A. 2007;**70**(1):7-18

[289] Kharbanda EO, Vazquez-Benitez G, Kunin-Batson A, Nordin JD, Olsen A, Romitti PA. Birth and early developmental screening outcomes associated with cannabis exposure during pregnancy. Journal of Perinatology. 2020;**40**(3):473-480

[290] Linn S, Schoenbaum SC, Monson RR, Rosner R, Stubblefield PC,

Ryan KJ. The association of marijuana use with outcome of pregnancy. American Journal of Public Health. 1983;**73**(10):1161-1164

[291] Petrangelo A, Czuzoj-Shulman N, Balayla J, Abenhaim HA. Cannabis abuse or dependence during pregnancy: A population-based cohort study on 12 million births. Journal of Obstetrics and Gynaecology Canada. 2019;**41**(5):623-630

[292] Warshak CR, Regan J, Moore B, Magner K, Kritzer S, Van Hook J. Association between marijuana use and adverse obstetrical and neonatal outcomes. Journal of Perinatology. 2015;**35**(12):991-995

[293] Brown SJ, Mensah FK, Ah Kit J, Stuart-Butler D, Glover K, Leane C, et al. Use of cannabis during pregnancy and birth outcomes in an Aboriginal birth cohort: A cross-sectional, population-based study. BMJ Open. 2016;**6**(2):e010286

[294] Chabarria KC, Racusin DA, Antony KM, Kahr M, Suter MA, Mastrobattista JM, et al. Marijuana use and its effects in pregnancy. American Journal of Obstetrics and Gynecology. 2016;**215**(4):506.e1-506.e7

[295] Corsi DJ, Walsh L, Weiss D, Hsu H, El-Chaar D, Hawken S, et al. Association between self-reported prenatal cannabis use and maternal, perinatal, and neonatal outcomes. Journal of the American Medical Association. 2019;**322**(2):145-152

[296] Crume TL, Juhl AL, Brooks-Russell A, Hall KE, Wymore E, Borgelt LM. Cannabis use during the perinatal period in a state with legalized recreational and medical marijuana: The association between maternal characteristics, breastfeeding patterns, and neonatal outcomes. The Journal of Pediatrics. 2018;**197**:90-96

[297] Hayatbakhsh MR, Flenady VJ, Gibbons KS, Kingsbury AM, Hurrion E, Mamun AA, et al. Birth outcomes associated with cannabis use before and during pregnancy. Pediatric Research. 2012;**71**(2):215-219

[298] Koto P, Allen VM, Fahey J, Kuhle S. Maternal cannabis use during pregnancy and maternal and neonatal outcomes: A retrospective cohort study. BJOG: An International Journal of Obstetrics and Gynaecology. 2022; DOI: 10.1111/1471-0528.17114. Online ahead of print

[299] Leemaqz SY, Dekker GA, McCowan LM, Kenny LC, Myers JE, Simpson NA, et al. Maternal marijuana use has independent effects on risk for spontaneous preterm birth but not other common late pregnancy complications. Reproductive Toxicology. 2016;**62**:77-86

[300] Luke S, Hutcheon J, Kendall T. Cannabis use in pregnancy in British Columbia and selected birth outcomes. Journal of Obstetrics and Gynaecology Canada. 2019;**41**(9):1311-1317

[301] Marchand G, Masoud AT, Govindan M, Ware K, King A, Ruther S, et al. Birth outcomes of neonates exposed to marijuana in utero: A systematic review and meta-analysis. JAMA Network Open. 2022;**5**(1):e2145653

[302] Nguyen VH, Harley KG. Prenatal cannabis use and infant birth outcomes in the pregnancy risk assessment monitoring system. The Journal of Pediatrics. 2021;**240**:87-93

[303] Sasso EB, Bolshakova M, Bogumil D, Johnson B, Komatsu E, Sternberg J, et al. Marijuana use and perinatal outcomes in obstetric patients at a safety net hospital. European

Journal of Obstetrics, Gynecology, and Reproductive Biology. 2021;**266**:36-41

[304] Shi Y, Zhu B, Liang D. The associations between prenatal cannabis use disorder and neonatal outcomes. Addiction. 2021;**116**(11):3069-3079

[305] Straub HL, Mou J, Drennan KJ, Pflugeisen BM. Maternal marijuana exposure and birth weight: An observational study surrounding recreational marijuana legalization. American Journal of Perinatology. 2021;**38**(1):65-75

[306] ElSohly MA, Feng S. delta 9-THC metabolites in meconium: Identification of 11-OH-delta 9-THC, 8 beta,11-diOH-delta 9-THC, and 11-nor-delta 9-THC-9-COOH as major metabolites of delta 9-THC. Journal of Analytical Toxicology. 1998;**22**(4):329-335

[307] ElSohly MA, Stanford DF, Murphy TP, Lester BM, Wright LL, Smeriglio VL, et al. Immunoassay and GC-MS procedures for the analysis of drugs of abuse in meconium. Journal of Analytical Toxicology. 1999;**23**(6):436-445

[308] Joya X, Pujadas M, Falcon M, Civit E, Garcia-Algar O, Vall O, et al. Gas chromatography-mass spectrometry assay for the simultaneous quantification of drugs of abuse in human placenta at 12th week of gestation. Forensic Science International. 2010;**196**(1-3):38-42

[309] Kim J, de Castro A, Lendoiro E, Cruz-Landeira A, Lopez-Rivadulla M, Concheiro M. Detection of in utero cannabis exposure by umbilical cord analysis. Drug Testing and Analysis. 2018;**10**(4):636-643

[310] Marchei E, Pellegrini M, Pacifici R, Palmi I, Lozano J, Garcia-Algar O, et al. Quantification of Delta9-tetrahydrocannabinol and its major metabolites in meconium by gas chromatographic-mass spectrometric assay: Assay validation and preliminary results of the "meconium project". Therapeutic Drug Monitoring. 2006;**28**(5):700-706

[311] Perez-Reyes M, Lipton MA, Timmons MC, Wall ME, Brine DR, Davis KH. Pharmacology of orally administered 9-tetrahydrocannabinol. Clinical Pharmacology and Therapeutics. 1973;**14**(1):48-55

[312] Baker T, Datta P, Rewers-Felkins K, Thompson H, Kallem RR, Hale TW. Transfer of inhaled cannabis into human breast milk. Obstetrics and Gynecology. 2018;**131**(5):783-788

[313] Moss MJ, Bushlin I, Kazmierczak S, Koop D, Hendrickson RG, Zuckerman KE, et al. Cannabis use and measurement of cannabinoids in plasma and breast milk of breastfeeding mothers. Pediatric Research. 2021;**90**(4):861-868

[314] Perez-Reyes M, Wall ME. Presence of delta9-tetrahydrocannabinol in human milk. The New England Journal of Medicine. 1982;**307**(13):819-820

[315] Sempio C, Wymore E, Palmer C, Bunik M, Henthorn TK, Christians U, et al. Detection of cannabinoids by LC-MS-MS and ELISA in breast milk. Journal of Analytical Toxicology. 2021;**45**(7):686-692

[316] Wymore EM, Palmer C, Wang GS, Metz TD, Bourne DWA, Sempio C, et al. Persistence of Δ-9-tetrahydrocannabinol in human breast milk. JAMA Pediatrics. 2021;**175**(6):632-634

[317] Behavioral Risk Factor Surveillance System (BRFSS) data. Colorado Department of Public Health and Environment. Available from:

https://marijuanahealthinfo.colorado.gov/health-data/behavioral-risk-factor-surveillance-system-brfss-data

[318] Aldington S, Williams M, Nowitz M, Weatherall M, Pritchard A, McNaughton A, et al. Effects of cannabis on pulmonary structure, function and symptoms. Thorax. 2007;**62**(12):1058-1063

[319] Bloom JW, Kaltenborn WT, Paoletti P, Camilli A, Lebowitz MD. Respiratory effects of non-tobacco cigarettes. British Medical Journal. 1987;**295**(6612):1516-1518

[320] Kempker JA, Honig EG, Martin GS. The effects of marijuana exposure on expiratory airflow. A study of adults who participated in the U.S. National Health and Nutrition Examination Study. Annals of the American Thoracic Society. 2015;**12**(2):135-141

[321] Macleod J, Robertson R, Copeland L, McKenzie J, Elton R, Reid P. Cannabis, tobacco smoking, and lung function: A cross-sectional observational study in a general practice population. The British Journal of General Practice. 2015;**65**(631):e89-e95

[322] Moore BA, Augustson EM, Moser RP, Budney AJ. Respiratory effects of marijuana and tobacco use in a U.S. sample. Journal of General Internal Medicine. 2005;**20**(1):33-37

[323] Morris MA, Jacobson SR, Kinney GL, Tashkin DP, Woodruff PG, Hoffman EA, et al. Marijuana use associations with pulmonary symptoms and function in tobacco smokers enrolled in the subpopulations and intermediate outcome measures in COPD study (SPIROMICS). Chronic Obstructive Pulmonary Disease. 2018;**5**(1):46-56

[324] Roth MD, Arora A, Barsky SH, Kleerup EC, Simmons M, Tashkin DP. Airway inflammation in young marijuana and tobacco smokers. American Journal of Respiratory and Critical Care Medicine. 1998;**157**(3 Pt 1):928-937

[325] Sherrill DL, Krzyzanowski M, Bloom JW, Lebowitz MD. Respiratory effects of non-tobacco cigarettes: A longitudinal study in general population. International Journal of Epidemiology. 1991;**20**(1):132-137

[326] Tashkin DP, Coulson AH, Clark VA, Simmons M, Bourque LB, Duann S, et al. Respiratory symptoms and lung function in habitual heavy smokers of marijuana alone, smokers of marijuana and tobacco, smokers of tobacco alone, and nonsmokers. The American Review of Respiratory Disease. 1987;**135**(1):209-216

[327] Taylor DR, Poulton R, Moffitt TE, Ramankutty P, Sears MR. The respiratory effects of cannabis dependence in young adults. Addiction. 2000;**95**(11):1669-1677

[328] Tashkin DP, Shapiro BJ, Frank IM. Acute pulmonary physiologic effects of smoked marijuana and oral 9 -tetrahydrocannabinol in healthy young men. The New England Journal of Medicine. 1973;**289**(7):336-341

[329] Tashkin DP, Shapiro BJ, Frank IM. Acute effects of smoked marijuana and oral delta9-tetrahydrocannabinol on specific airway conductance in asthmatic subjects. The American Review of Respiratory Disease. 1974;**109**(4):420-428

[330] Tashkin DP, Shapiro BJ, Lee YE, Harper CE. Effects of smoked marijuana in experimentally induced asthma. The American Review of Respiratory Disease. 1975;**112**(3):377-386

[331] Dean D, Passalacqua KD, Oh SM, Aaron C, Van Harn MG, King A. Pediatric cannabis single-substance exposures reported to the michigan poison center from 2008-2019 after medical marijuana legalization. The Journal of Emergency Medicine. 2021;**60**(6):701-708

[332] Myran DT, Cantor N, Finkelstein Y, Pugliese M, Guttmann A, Jesseman R, et al. Unintentional pediatric cannabis exposures after legalization of recreational cannabis in canada. JAMA Network Open. 2022;**5**(1):e2142521

[333] Onders B, Casavant MJ, Spiller HA, Chounthirath T, Smith GA. Marijuana exposure among children younger than six years in the United States. Clinical Pediatrics (Phila). 2016;**55**(5):428-436

[334] Shi Y, Liang D. The association between recreational cannabis commercialization and cannabis exposures reported to the US National Poison Data System. Addiction. 2020;**115**(10):1890-1899

[335] Thomas AA, Dickerson-Young T, Mazor S. Unintentional pediatric marijuana exposures at a tertiary care children's hospital in Washington State: A retrospective review. Pediatric Emergency Care. 2021;**37**(10):e594-e5e8

[336] Wang GS, Banerji S, Contreras AE, Hall KE. Marijuana exposures in Colorado, reported to regional poison centre, 2000-2018. Injury Prevention. 2020;**26**(2):184-186

[337] Wang GS, Le Lait MC, Deakyne SJ, Bronstein AC, Bajaj L, Roosevelt G. Unintentional pediatric exposures to marijuana in Colorado, 2009-2015. JAMA Pediatrics. 2016;**170**(9):e160971

[338] Wang GS, Roosevelt G, Heard K. Pediatric marijuana exposures in a medical marijuana state. JAMA Pediatrics. 2013;**167**(7):630-633

[339] Wang GS, Roosevelt G, Le Lait MC, Martinez EM, Bucher-Bartelson B, Bronstein AC, et al. Association of unintentional pediatric exposures with decriminalization of marijuana in the United States. Annals of Emergency Medicine. 2014;**63**(6):684-689

[340] Whitehill JM, Dilley JA, Brooks-Russell A, Terpak L, Graves JM. Edible cannabis exposures among children: 2017-2019. Pediatrics. 2021;**147**(4):e2020019893

[341] Whitehill JM, Harrington C, Lang CJ, Chary M, Bhutta WA, Burns MM. Incidence of pediatric cannabis exposure among children and teenagers aged 0 to 19 years before and after medical marijuana legalization in Massachusetts. JAMA Network Open. 2019;**2**(8):e199456

[342] Breault HJ. Five years with 5 million child-resistant containers. Clinical Toxicology. 1974;7(1):91-95

[343] Clarke A, Walton WW. Effect of safety packaging on aspirin ingestion by children. Pediatrics. 1979;**63**(5):687-693

[344] Rodgers GB. The effectiveness of child-resistant packaging for aspirin. Archives of Pediatrics & Adolescent Medicine. 2002;**156**(9):929-933

[345] The Health Effects of Cannabis and Cannabinoids: The Current State of Evidence and Recommendations for Research. Washington, DC: The National Academies Collection: Reports Funded by National Institutes of Health; 2017